Premature Ejaculation

The Ultimate Guide on How to Overcome PE, Have Better Sex and Improve the Power of Your Sexual Energy. Learn How to Get Complete Control over Ejaculation and Last Longer in Bed

Louie Holmes

Table of Contents

Introduction

If you're reading this ebook, you already know what it can be like to occasionally ejaculate sooner than you and your partner would like. Sure, it's annoying. You're embarrassed, self-conscious, and worried you haven't pleased her. But is it a real problem? As frustrating as it is, coming too quickly every now and then isn't usually a cause for concern. In fact, it happens to most guys from time to time.

But what if you consistently ejaculate too soon? What if intercourse typically only lasts about a minute, sometimes mere seconds? What if you find yourself constantly feeling ashamed, anxious, and stressed out by even the thought of sex because you know you can't last? What if you've never known any other way?

If this sounds like you, you could have premature ejaculation. You're not alone. Premature ejaculation, or PE, is the most common type of sexual dysfunction a man can have. Some experts estimate that up to 30 percent of men have premature ejaculation but you wouldn't know it from talking to your friends. To say that it's tough to talk about premature ejaculation is an understatement. Most guys don't want to admit that

1

they've got any kind of sexual problem, especially one as sensitive as ejaculating too soon.

What You Can Learn From This Book

This book teaches you exactly what you need to know and do to last longer in bed. It offers a proven step by step solution to premature ejaculation. It offers a way to be free from anxiety about ejaculation and have rock steady confidence sexually. It opens a gateway to great sex.

This programme set out in this book is unique. You will not find anything else like it.

Is This Book For Me?

This book is right for you:

■   If you have suffered long term with serious premature ejaculation to the point where it has interfered with your fulfilment in sex and relationships.

■   If you have recently developed premature ejaculation and don't understand why.

■ If you have never lasted particularly long but would like to last longer.

■ If you are feeling pressured by your partner to "do better" in bed.

■ If you have a good sex life and good staying power but you'd like to be even better.

How to Use this Book

This book has been designed specifically to help you get rid of your issues and problems with premature ejaculation. The tips, information, exercises and techniques mentioned in this book are all tried and tested. They have been able to show the most desirable results for many people who wanted to get rid of their problems with premature ejaculation and improve their sex life.

All the instructions for exercises and techniques provided in this book are based on real life results, and yet we are not doctors or medical experts who can certify their effectiveness. This book is a result of thorough practical research and theoretical studies. The best way to make your efforts more effective is by adding a good deal of confidence in yourself.

The rest will follow with paying attention to the instructions provided through this book. You have to display a good deal of patience and perseverance, as the results may not be immediate, and might take some time to show.

One of the most important things to learn through this book is how you can understand your body better, and read the responses in the correct way to make them work for you.

You will notice that there are a number of techniques mentioned in this book. However, the idea is to learn more about your body (the concerned parts of your body) and understand how everything works and how you can control it better. This will undoubtedly show you great results, and improve your abilities in sex.

This is why I have provided a huge deal of information about the causes of premature ejaculation. Again, the results are not something that you can hope to achieve in a couple of days. You need to be able to understand everything with relation to how your mind behaves, and how your body reacts to the sensory responses.

If you want long term and stable results, the timeframe we are looking at is around 3 weeks. However, the results can be seen within a single week as well, depending on your abilities. To see the best results, you will have to maintain a positive attitude at all times, and confidence is your strongest weapon. Never think about premature ejaculation as a problem. It is nothing but your body being extra fine tuned for reproduction. You have a better reproductive system that most of the others around you.

Finally, make sure to start with the first chapter, go through each chapter closely, in proper sequence. And at the same time, taking notes while going through each of the chapters is also a good practice. Take clear notes, and go over the whole book a few times to ensure you are aware of everything that has been mentioned in this book. Take it as a course, and try to check on yourself whether you have followed the instructions clearly.

General Disclaimer

This book and the information it contains for the readers has been seen to be very effective. However, there are a few things that need important consideration here. First of all, you should not expect the results to present themselves over a couple of days. For the best results, one must go on with the exercises and tips for around 3 weeks.

The success solely depends on the efforts the reader has put in, and also on the constitution of their body systems to a great deal of time. At the same time, we are no doctors or medical experts who can vouch for the results.

Chapter 1: Understanding Premature Ejaculation

The most vital part of this book is understanding what premature ejaculation is, which is where we will start. To be able to understand clearly how everything works and whether you are doing things the right way, you need to go through some basic information with relation to your body and the ejaculation process.

The most important thing to understand here is that you must be aware of how things work, and why they work that way. Only then will you be able to completely understand premature ejaculation and see the best results in sorting this issue out.

This chapter is what the whole book is built on, and it therefore becomes very important for you to go through each and every point discussed here in the best possible way.

What is Premature EJaculation?

You might be surprised to hear this, but premature ejaculation is something that a lot of us are seen to suffer from. It is almost 20 to 40% of the male population who think they suffer from premature ejaculation at some point in their lives. And this is nothing strange. Most of us have a very wrong concept about PE. In the real sense of it, when your reproductive system is extra fine tuned, you tend to be able to ejaculate very easily, over very little time.

Thus, this only means that you enjoy a sound reproductive system, and should not be ashamed of your issues with premature ejaculation at any point of time.

There is nothing that is wrong medically with premature ejaculation. It has a lot to do with your state of mind, and what you think about it. Quite a bit depends on the conditions and the situations that you are in as well. And the fact that you think you might experience premature ejaculation may not be true at all, as people have different ideas about this. Since you are reading this book, let's make sure you have a clear idea on this so that we can approach it in a much better way.

There are diverse ideas on what premature ejaculation is, and these ideas vary a lot with respect to people who have these ideas on their minds. Some people would consider the amount of time they can last before they come to judge whether premature ejaculation might be a problem for them. Others might check on how many strokes would exactly make them ejaculate. And there are a number of definitions and views on premature ejaculation as well.

To understand more about premature ejaculation, you first need to understand how your body and the ejaculation process work. You might imagine that ejaculation—the release of seminal fluid from your body—is limited to your penis, testicles, and other reproductive organs, but you'd be wrong. In fact, your nervous system plays a key role.

Some parts of sexual arousal fall within parasympathetic nervous system responses and other processes fall within sympathetic. The sympathetic nervous sys-tem controls your body's stress-related functions like the "fight or flight" response, which allowed your cave-man ancestors to battle or escape dangerous predators. (These days, you're more likely to rely on your fight-or-flight response before a big meeting with your boss.) Your parasympathetic nervous system controls your "rest and digest" response—lower blood pressure, a slower heartbeat, and other functions related to relaxation.

The process begins when you're sexually aroused, often but not always from the direct physical stimulation of your penis during touching, rubbing, oral sex, or intercourse, for example. Your brain responds by sending signals to your lower spinal cord. You get an erection, thanks to your parasympathetic nervous system. As a result, the muscles in your prostate gland, seminal vesicles (both of which produce seminal fluid), and vas deferens (the tube that connects the testicles to the urethra) contract rhythmically, moving semen through those glands and the urethra and out of your body, a process controlled by the sympathetic nervous system. An orgasm is the sensation of pleasure you feel during ejaculation.

Premature ejaculation occurs when this process takes place earlier than you and your partner would like on a consistent basis.

So the whole point of considering premature ejaculation is to satisfy your partner, isn't it? It is ideally not about masturbation, but about real penetration and sex. So, why not consider premature ejaculation with whether you are able to ejaculate after you have satisfied your partner or not? Thus, it ultimately comes down to whether your partner gets to see orgasm before you ejaculate.

In other words, it means that you would want to cure premature ejaculation based on the sexual satisfaction levels of your particular partner.

How Does It Affect You

Disagreements aside, in general, chronic, lifelong premature ejaculation involves three main issues:

- How long you last before you orgasm

- Whether or not you can delay ejaculation

- Negative personal consequences

Let's break those issues down one by one...

You don't last long.

Think you have premature ejaculation because you can't keep going for hours on end? Forget about what you've seen in movies or heard about in the locker room. Most guys can actually only have intercourse for an average of about two to five minutes before ejaculating. For men with premature ejaculation, though, that's an eternity—most can only last about a minute or less before they come.

Researchers have devised a system called *Intravaginal Ejaculatory Latency Time (IELT),* which measures how long a man can have intercourse before he ejaculates. Different researchers have found different times, but most report that men with premature ejaculation typically last somewhere between 15 and 60 seconds.

Many guys with premature ejaculation don't even make it to penetration. They orgasm during frottage (heavy petting), they orgasm with any direct manual stimu-lation, and they orgasm during oral stimulation. As a result, most men with premature ejaculation consider these activities off-limits, so they have a hard time enjoying the full spectrum of sexual possibility. They also have a difficult time explaining why it's so hard for them to receive sexual stimulation, which can often leave their female partners feeling confused and less engaged.

You can't hold back.

The old *"think about baseball"* trick doesn't work for guys with Premature ejaculation. They can't control or delay ejaculation at, or shortly after, penetration whether they want to or not. Of course, all men have a point of what I call *"ejaculatory inevitability"* during sex when they can't hold back from an orgasm, no matter what. And all men have an *"ejaculatory threshold,"* which is the amount of stimulation they can experience before reaching this *"point of no return."* That threshold is lower in guys with premature ejaculation, and their point of ejaculatory inevitability arrives much more quickly.

Women, on the other hand, don't experience ejaculatory inevitability—they can *"lose"* an orgasm even as it's happening. When you realize that many women are unfamiliar with the concepts of ejaculatory inevitability and ejaculatory threshold, it makes sense that they want to get their guy as turned on as possible. But that's the wrong approach for men with Premature ejaculation. In some ways, one of the worst things a woman can say to man with premature ejaculation is to ask him to *"wait"* to have his orgasm. In fact, the stress of being told to wait until you're ready is likely to speed up ejaculatory inevitability, as you'll learn later. All this can make it really difficult to bring a woman to orgasm through intercourse. Because each woman is different—and her ability to orgasm can fluctuate—you can't judge whether you have premature ejaculation based on how long it takes her to come. But, in general, men with premature ejaculation can't last long enough to satisfy a woman during vaginal inter-course. No wonder many men with premature ejaculation are constantly worried about sexual failure.

Premature ejaculation affects your life.

I don't have to tell you that those first two issues—not being able to last long enough and not being able to hold back—do nothing to inspire sexual confidence. Instead, they can trigger a whole range of negative emotions in men with Premature ejaculation: You might feel angry and frustrated with yourself, insecure and anxious about your sex life, embarrassed, worried about your relationship, or a combination of these.

Many men with premature ejaculation worry that their partners will think they're sexually lazy or selfish and some women who don't understand premature ejaculation may indeed think that. The irony is that guys with premature ejaculation tend to be extremely sensitive lovers but are incapable of putting that intent into action. But being constantly hung up on delaying your orgasm can make it difficult for you to enjoy sex, and you may end up avoiding women, relationships, and sexual situations as a result. I frequently hear from women who don't know that their partner is dealing with premature ejaculation and think something else is wrong with the relationship. They wonder why their partners are depressed, distant, or avoiding sex. And premature ejaculation doesn't just affect the woman in your life: You might even retreat from your male friendships because you feel like less of a man when hearing other guys talk about sex.

All this can make you feel really alone, like you can't talk to anyone about it. premature ejaculation can make you feel sexually immature and out of control, and it's easy to beat yourself up about it if you don't understand what's happening and why. Later on, I'll show you how to cope with these types of emotions so you can feel more confident.

Chapter 2: Causes of Premature Ejaculation

Believe it or not, premature ejaculation wasn't always considered a problem infact, it used to be something to strive for! Hundreds of thousands of years ago, the premature ejaculator would have been considered the superior male because he could fertilize a woman more quickly. That allowed him to have sex with more women and father more children, winning the "sperm wars" and earning his place at the head of his tribe.

It also helped his family thrive. Cavemen and women weren't exactly retiring to a swanky honeymoon suite to get it on: most sex was had outdoors, where animal predators could easily make the couple into a tasty snack. This added risk contributed to anxiety, causing the man to ejaculate even earlier. Yet men who finished faster were valued because shorter sex meant reduced exposure to danger. In primitive times, there was likely little to no awareness of the female orgasm, so coming quickly probably wasn't considered a problem for either party. We've all heard the phrase "survival of the fittest," but in sexual terms it was all about survival of the quickest.

This trait, some experts believe, was passed down from generation to generation, making what we now call premature ejaculation an evolutionary benefit. (Although most of us would view it as an evolutionary drawback.) But today's PE-ers also appear to have inherited our forefathers' sensitivity to environmental stressors, like loud noises. In this case, though, the culprit is more likely to be a honking horn than a growling saber-toothed tiger. I've even had new fathers tell me that just hearing their baby cry from the other room when they're having sex almost always triggers ejaculation!

These days, our knowledge of female sexual pleasure and our ability to couple safely and privately means that premature ejaculation is less of an evolutionary benefit than a flaw. **So why do some many men still have Premature ejaculation?**

In some cultures, premature ejaculation is said to be caused by everything from "weak blood" or "loose nerves" to cold weather or stress. Sounds ridiculous, right? But the real causes of premature ejaculation aren't so easy to identify.

Over the years, a number of different causes of premature ejaculation have been suggested. And while there may be some truth to some of them, none of these causes appear to be the only reason a man develops remature ejaculation. Let's take a look at some of the more common theories.

Physical Causes

High blood pressure

Most people who are suffering from high blood pressure experience little if any symptoms at all, but the effect which this condition can have on your sex life if often significant and signs of sexual difficulty can sound a warning bell.

The effect of high blood pressure is to damage the lining of your blood vessels and to cause hardening of your arteries so that your heart is forced to work harder to pump blood around your body. This in turn raises the pressure in your arteries. In addition, the damage to your arteries results in a general reduction in the flow of blood throughout your body.

As far as men are concerned this general reduction in blood flow also means a reduced flow of blood to the penis and difficulty in both achieving and maintaining an erection. It also means that, even when you can achieve and maintain an erection, high blood pressure can create problems with ejaculation. For the majority of men the appearance of the first signs of sexual dysfunction is very worrying and concern that, having happened for the first time, the problem might well reappear. This leads some men to avoid sex so that not only does the event cause them distress, but it also often generates problems in their relationship with their sexual partner.

In the case of women the effect of high blood pressure is not as clearly defined and, at this time, has not been well researched. We do know however that high blood pressure causes a lower flow of blood to the vagina, leading to lower sexual desire and arousal, vaginal dryness and problems in achieving orgasm. As with men, most women find this event very worrying and will again shy away from sex, putting their relationship with their sexual partner under strain.

There are many simple natural solutions to hypertension. This involves the use of effective nutritional supplements in the right dosages thereby helping to prevent and reverse it. It is the number one modifiable risk factor for stroke. It also contributes to heart attacks, heart failure, kidney failure and atherosclerosis (fatty buildups in arteries). In some cases it can also result to blindness.

Diabetes

A diabetic patient whether male or female is bound to be restricted to nutritious and energizing diet. As a consequence of having poor food to avoid hypoglycemia, the total system loses its vigor which includes the genital function also.

Men with diabetes have to face the daily struggles with their ailment. Along with all other complications, diabetics are likely to contend with sexual problems causing to affect their bed scenes and seeking for impotence remedies. Hyperglycemic condition with diabetics does affect adversely the nervous system, which in turn creates problems in bed relation. Men with diabetes are more vulnerable than the women partner. Very often a small physical problem can snowball into a big concern with less impulses of libido enhancer. The active role of male is more emphatic than that of female, although equal role is needed in bed relation. The major problems are 4 in number.

■ Inability to play sex game, of course to satisfy the female partner is a serious problem.

■ Pre-ejaculation or quick ejaculation of semen is also a problem for men diabetics.

■ Anxiety due to no confidence in starting the game.

■ Resultant depression of mind with complex feelings.

However, one should not imagine any or every other problem related to sex organ to be exclusively due to diabetic condition. Some other reasons may also be accountable. Diabetes alone cannot be the sole cause for such problems.

Drinking

In many comic television shows, drinking an excessive amount of alcohol makes a man able to approach the woman of is dreams and proposition her. In both the comedy and in real life, this is most often met by a drink in the face, but for many men, having a few drinks lowers inhibitions and makes them more willing to experiment in bed. However, there's a very fine line between lowering inhibitions... and lowering everything else!

Alcohol has a detrimental effect on male sexual health by suppressing testosterone and killing sperm. Alcohol also has a 'feminizing' effect on men; it creates man boobs, makes the body store more fat around the hips and reduces chest hair because alcohol as more estrogen in it and it lowers testosterone levels too. Alcohol has also been found to shrink the testes of men.

All of these physical factors also work against a longer period before ejaculation. Not only do drunken men tend to 'cum' faster because they aren't bothering to control themselves, but they have lost many of the natural safeguards of their body such as testosterone and normal sized organs.

However, like most things, the bad things will only happen if you overdo it all of the time. Many men have found that a moderate amount of alcohol improves their performance because of lowered inhibitions and a more numb feeling. However, this doesn't help sensation and a lot of the drinks that men indulge in are not the ones needed to stay on the good side of the line (ie. Men tend to drink a lot of beer which ruins sexual encounters where instead they should be having a glass of wine over dinner to help the encounter). It's a very fine line and one that most men ignore in favor of drinking it up and falling into a stupor!

If you want to use alcohol to occasionally give you a boost in longevity or to last longer in bed, then opt for a romantic dinner with wine, not for beer and you'll find that you'll perform better-but don't use alcohol as a crutch either. If you have a problem with premature ejaculation, drinking any kind of alcohol will, over the long run, make the problem worse, not better.

Excessive Masturbation

Excessive masturbation can be easily compared with an addiction. Men practicing it are aware that they are doing something wrong and something dangerous for their health, but they simply can't stop. There are also cases of men who are not informed about the bad effects of over masturbation and continue in this ill practice until they start experiencing the consequences.

Masturbation is considered by some experts healthy for someone's sex life. It begins in puberty years when a teenager gradually discovers his sexuality. It might accompany a man up to older ages, especially in times when he is lonely. It's nothing wrong with it as long as it stays within normal limits. The tricky part is that what is considered normal in what concerns the limits differs from individual to individual. The only number that is commonly agreed on is 3: a man shouldn't ejaculate more than three times a week.

Over masturbation practice is very harmful for one's health and its bad effects are devastating. The physical consequences are indeed serious, but the psychological effects are the ones that really put a man down. Excessive masturbation causes weak nerves, muscles and swelling in the internal organs which causes problems like premature ejaculation, nightfall and even erectile dysfunction, low sperm count and low sperm motility. Weakening of PC muscles due to excessive masturbation is the biggest cause of premature ejaculation and nightfall in a male. PC muscles control ejaculation whether voluntary or involuntary, but due to frequent masturbation body loses control over these muscles and thus cannot control ejaculation too.

Excessive masturbation can stop you from living a normal life next to the woman you love. It needs to be cut down completely because the price you have to pay for indulging in pleasure all by yourself is too high. The bad effects on your body will become so serious, unless you treat them, that you won't even be able to enjoy the pleasure you want to produce yourself, not to mention pleasure with a woman.

Prostatitis

The prostate gland is a vital component of your sexual equipment. If it's inflamed or enlarged, called prostatitis, it can easily make you more sensitive to stimulation and more likely to cum at a moment's notice. If you're very sensitive down there or have trouble peeing, see your physician for a referral to a urologist to check you out. And if you're taking any prescription drugs, discuss sexual side effects that you could be experiencing.

Fortunately, there are some natural remedies that can improve your prostate health. Take Saw Palmetto and Pygeum daily, two natural herbs you can get at the health food store. Research has shown these supplements can help your prostate significantly.

While we're on the subject, there are some other common substances which can inflame your prostate and make you more sensitive to cuming. Can you guess what they are? Right, I'm talking about caffeine, nicotine, and alcohol. If you smoke and drink coffee and alcohol, you would be well advised to avoid them during this program.

Low serotonin content in your system

One of the other reasons why you might be seeing premature ejaculation issues is the low serotonin content in your system. Most people who experience from severe premature ejaculation see their bodies devoid of the right quantity of serotonin, which disables them of being able to control their urge to ejaculate. This can be understood when you consider the drugs and medicines that contain serotonin and how they affect your sex drive.

For example, consider the anti depressants (SSRIs). Over consumption, and even a regular course of such medicine, will make it quite a tough task for you to feel the urge to ejaculate. This is exactly why anti depressants often lower down your sex drive and make you lose interest in love making.

Psychological Causes

Stress

Have you ever stopped to think just how much your level of stress is affecting your daily life? You may not have even let that thought cross your mind before, but the truth is that being stressed out has more effects on your day to day happenings and activities than you may ever realize. For instance, you may not know this, but being stressed out and frustrated is one of the main causes of premature ejaculation. With people losing their jobs everyday and the natural occurrences of life that just seem to pile up on top of you sometimes, stress levels can go through the roof if you are not careful and do not take control of them early on.

First of all, lets look at how stress can lead to an inability to control an orgasm and sustain a healthy sexual experience. The mind is the most powerful sexual organ that you have. Your brain controls whether or not you become aroused or even interested in sex, your ability to have an erection, and your ability to control your orgasms. Frustration and stress about something trivial can put a stop to all of these functions. The brain gets clouded when you are frustrated and it tends to only focus on the thing that you are stressed out about. If you can just learn to let these stresses go then you will be able to experience the fullness of sexual performance and delight without any hindrances.

Stressing about an issue in your life can make you unable to think about anything else other than that event, so during the act of intercourse, you will have an extremely hard time focusing on controlling your orgasm. Your mind is what makes it possible for you to be able to relax and control your ejaculatory functions. If your brain is cluttered with stress you will not be able to control your sexual functions in this way because all you will be thinking about is your frustrations and problems with anxiety.

One of the best things that you can do is simply breathe deeply and let your frustrations go. Go outside and go for a walk or maybe a bike ride. Getting out into the outside world can be one of the best ways for you to experience a new and fresh view on your life as it relates to the big world around you. There are so many people who have so many problems and stresses just like you do and when you begin to see this is when you begin to realize that yours aren't so bad. The moment that you realize that your stress doesn't have to be a problem is the moment that it stops being a problem. Releasing your stress means you will be able to enjoy sex with the fullness that you were meant to enjoy it with. You are far less likely to experience problems with premature ejaculation when you have a clear head and a clean conscious.

Anxiety

It seems that anxiety and premature ejaculation go hand in hand all too often. In men, anxiety is another contributing factor to what causes premature ejaculation; this is perhaps the driving force behind sexual dysfunction in general. It begins from the worry of not being capable to satisfy the spouse. When you are very nervous, you may not be capable to take your spouse to orgasm. Unfortunately, there are a number of reasons a person could experience anxiety. Are you comfortable being naked in front of anyone? If the answer is *"NO"* then you'll probably feel nervous in front of your partner. Being anxious during sex because of bad past experiences can also lead to questioning your sexual ability the next time you have sex. This turns into a self-destructive cycle; bad experience begets more bad experiences.

When you undress and a woman grabs your penis it may cause you to prematurely ejaculate, when a woman gives you oral sex it may also very quickly make you want to ejaculate.

You may experience something called penetration anxiety, when you are about to penetrate your woman you get this feeling of anxiety, either you can't keep your erection strong enough to enter your woman or you prematurely ejaculate as soon as you enter her.

Learning to relax and treating anxiety is perhaps one of the biggest factors to overcome. There are a variety of techniques that can help in treating anxiety; however realizing you actually are experiencing anxiety during sex is the first step. When the sensations during your sexual experience began to surface, immediately change your focus to something else, like your breathing. Is it erratic? Or are you breathing deep and slow?

Lack of Experience

In our society, for the most part, sex is a private experience because it's a taboo subject. We hide our insecurities, make rude jokes, and don't talk about it openly. Too many of us obsess about when to make the first move, or how to initiate with a long-time partner instead of joyously enjoying verbal foreplay. No wonder so many of us build up the anxieties and tensions we talked about earlier that can cause premature ejaculation.

We're not taught that sex is communion between souls expressing their basic nature through the divine gift of bodies. Few of us learn to play these instruments in harmony to produce amazing ecstasy. Where do we learn that sex is an energy exchange between conscious beings who want to both give and receive pleasure? When you're desired and accepted for who you are without big expectations about how you need to perform, then you can relax and let nature take it's sexual course. That's partly why the solutions in this ebook requires "partnering" with your lovers. This means being aware of your needs and reactions, talking honestly about them, honoring those of your partner, and playing together as equals. Instead of 'doing' your partner, you'll need to do new-age things like sharing together. (Come on, don't gag, be open to dramatic change, buddy. You're here because you chose to become different, right?)

Different partners have different sexual responses. There are women who could cum very quickly, but most need lots of stimulation. Myself, I always like lots of touching all over my body. So who's responsible for seeing that each partner gets the things that bring them the most pleasure? We each are fully responsible. Partnering means speaking your needs and honoring those of your partners. If we do anything else, we set up the dynamics that produce stress, mystery, and tension - a surefire prescription for blowing your wad unexpectedly.

If you're single and searching for a partner to satisfy sexually, this whole view of sex as communion may sound even more challenging than finding someone willing to jump in the sack. (Please, no paper bag jokes.) If you expect that you alone will be able to satisfy any woman without their cooperation, you're laboring under a big delusion, friend. Drop the whole concept that it's your job alone to satisfy your partner. This is a mutual dance and that's the way most women love it. Later, I'll show you how to broach this delicate subject with potential partners that will make you seem more desirable to them, not less.

The Mind

Without a doubt, the mind is a powerful sex organ. We all attract what we focus on. For example, if your whole attention is on your genitals, than your sexual energy has no where else to go but out that little hole in your little head. If you're intent on the goal of giving your partner an orgasm, then you're likely to attract one too soon - namely one of your own. Case histories of psychological reasons for premature ejaculation abound.

This approach is the solution so that you learn to enjoy sex even more while managing ejaculation. The mind's tricks - goals you're totally absorbed in or pervading mental images - get in the way of you tuning into the present moment. With these consuming internal distractions, how can you truly appreciate what's happening now? Instead, you need to shift your attention to your senses, your whole body, feelings and sensations - all the sources of pleasure imaginable. Lots more about this later.

The essence of this ebook is to get out of your head and into your body. Relax and stay in the moment, tuning into those wonderful feelings emanating from your sensitive places. Drop all your standards and goals and just ride the wave of energy. Don't push yourself or your partner for the Big O. When you learn to surf your sexual energy without attempting to control the outcome, you'll be able to go with the flow in a loose and natural way indefinitely.

Deeper Causes

Antisexual Childhood Messages

Among the most common deeper emotional problems we see in people with sexual disorders is guilt or shame about sexual pleasure. These are left- overs from old "messages" that sex is disgusting, sinful, and harmful which are transmitted to children by some puritanical families, schools, and churches.

Such early antisexual "programming" tends to remain with a person into his adult life and will put a damper on his sexuality even if he no longer believes this old propaganda intellectually, and even if he is not fully aware that he harbors these feelings.

A troubled family environment

Some people still carry emotional scars from growing up in neurotic families, and that is another source from the past which can lead to sexual difficulties. Rather than buffering their children from the stresses of the world as they should, some immature parents use their children as pawns in their fights with each other. Others, who themselves have emotional problems, lay their depression on their kids. Some mothers and fathers even act out their own craziness by behaving in an inappropriately sexually seductive or competitive manner with their child. Kids from such troubled families grow up with distorted ideas of sex, love, and marriage, and may have difficulties establishing normal romantic and sexual relationships when they grow up.

Still other parents, with sexual hang-ups of their own, stunt their children's sexual development by punishing them harshly for masturbating, or by threatening them with dire warnings at any display of their normal sexual feelings or curiosity. This gives kids the idea that they are bad if they enjoy sex and sets them up to feel guilty and anxious anytime they get aroused for the rest of their lives.

If you grew up in an unhealthy family environment, there is no point in getting angry at your mother or father. Parents do the best they can, but their own limitations may have resulted in their emotionally abusing you when you were an impressionable kid, to the detriment of your later sex life. There is also nothing to be gained by feeling sorry for yourself. Just get on with your life. Fortunately, the damage can most often be repaired, but only if you take responsibility for doing so for yourself.

Consider the theory of evolution

This will loudly point out at the same fact. Ejaculation was meant for procreation, and the sooner, the better. However, in men, there are a lot of other factors involved as well. For example, the responsiveness of the nervous system varies from man to man. And the nervous system is something that controls sex drive and ejaculation to a great extent.

The saddest part is, the more responsive your nervous system is, the quicker are you going to experience ejaculation. Consider the fact that young males are more likely to see premature ejaculation than older males. This is simply because of the responsiveness of the nervous system of the younger males. The ability to last longer comes with age, naturally, as the nervous system loses its efficiency gradually.

Thus, the quicker you ejaculate, the better your nervous system is, and this comes with your DNA, which is hereditary. However, this can easily be controlled according to your requirements if your approach is correct and you know how the systems work to understand how to use them better.

Chapter 3: Understanding Sexual Arousal

Everyone experienced sexual arousal differently because everyone has different preference to how they response sexually. Most commonly everyone get arouse from kissing and touching one another.

There are numerous nerve endings on the mouth and lips that provide sensual feeling and erotic pleasure when kissed. Kissing provide intimacy between both partners in which an individual feels good kissing someone as well as an individual feels good receiving a kiss.

Touching is also an important sense of arousal because an entire body can respond sexually to touching. Touching does not always have to be directed to the genital area to achieve arousal. Different people prefer different type of touching and some people prefer touching on the breast and nipple to get sexually aroused and other prefer touching and kissing all over the body before touching the genital.

Everyone also have different experience to sexual response from different method of stimulation. Some people get excited very quickly to certain stimulation and others may not feel the same way. The ability to get excited quickly during stimulation or sexual activity also has to do with age. When people get older the ability to get aroused and excited also take longer to happen but people continue to enjoy sexual activity in the old age.

Almost everyone experience orgasm after the excitement phase in response to sexual arousal. However as people get older the ability to experience orgasm may take longer to achieve and others may continue to experience orgasm less frequently and others may not be able to achieve orgasm at all. For older people that are able to achieve orgasm the experience are usually less intense and for older men the period after orgasm are lengthen for several hours or days before they are able to get sexually arouse or experience the next orgasm.

Men tend to forget that women are sexual creatures and that they love sex just as much as men. If you know this already, then it will be easier for you to learn how to sexually arouse a woman much easily and effectively.

A man who knows how to sexually arouse a woman has got something that the majority of man lacks and probably has a better sex life than most.

Phases of Sexual Arousal in Humans

Sensual Touch

"The fingertips are among the most reactive erogenous zones during arousal. Your heavy breathing cleanses carbon dioxide from the blood and alters the ionic balance of bodily fluids. The result is an increase in nerve activity and

excitation, which results in tingling at the skin's surface—particularly at the fingertips." — From *Sex Geeks*

Physical affection may be the most powerful of all love languages, and we have come to associate intimate touch with deep commitment. Women rate affection as one of the most important components of a loving relationship.

Plus, researchers have found that couples who caress one another experience a reduction in stress hormones, blood pressure, and blood sugar alongside an increase in oxytocin levels, improved pulmonary functioning, and heightened immunity. On top of the purported health benefits, being touched by a loved one also feels great!

Sensual touch is an extension of loving touch and different from therapeutic touch. You don't need to work out the knots in her back or soothe his aching neck during an erotic encounter. Instead, your touch is intended for mutual pleasure, relaxation, and connection, and it may or may not lead to further sex play. Unfortunately, many couples allow their erotic touch to taper off as their relationship progresses, and women often complain that their lovers do not touch or hug them in nonsexual situations.

This is a shame, as intimate touch is not just a precursor to sex but is related to higher levels of relationship satisfaction. Learning to touch your lover's entire body is a simple way to boost your happiness and ignite your sex life, so take some time to slow down and explore your bodies in their entirety without rushing to the genitals for instant gratification.

Massage Techniques

The sensual massage techniques that follow will have your lover's body writhing in pleasure and impassioned desire. Before you begin, make sure the room is a comfortable temperature and your partner is relaxed, whether that means sitting in a chair or lying on the bed. Make it interesting by giving her a blindfold to wear. You can take turns massaging each other, or dedicate an entire session to worshipping your lover's body alone.

■ *Spider pulls* are the perfect way to draw awareness and blood to the surface of her skin. Start with your fingers outstretched and the pads of your fingertips resting gently against her skin. Slowly and gently pull all five fingers together into the center with the lightest touch possible.

■ *Raindrops* produce a tingling sensation as you gently flutter the pads of your fingertips along his most sensitive regions. Start with his spine, underarms, shoulder blades, and butt cheeks.

■ *Finger stripes* allow you to draw erotic energy to a focused area of her body. Cover all five fingers in oil and run them in a straight line down the backs of her thighs, inner arms, or abdomen. Then retrace your path using your middle knuckles.

■ *Palm circles* get the blood flowing to all the right places. Just be sure to cover your hands in a light massage oil before circling them over his chest, abs, and hips.

■ *Figure eights* allow you to explore her body with large sweeping sensations. Use two wet fingers to trace loops of figure-eight patterns along her collarbone, arms, and the sides of her breasts.

■   *Tongue trails* offer a reminder that you don't need your hands to give a sensual massage. Trace your tongue all around his hot spots, alternating between a pointed tip and a wide, flat tongue.

■   *The body slide* is an advanced technique common in high-end massage parlors. Your lover lies on his stomach and you slide your entire body down the full length of his backside. You'll need to slather yourselves in oil for this one!

■   *Awakening touch* uses only the backs of your fingernails. This activates the nerve endings, referred to as the tactile corpuscles, that are most sensitive to light touch and are primed for heightened pleasure, as they don't interpret pain.

■   *Temperature* play can be highly erotic as you shift between breathing warm air against the skin with a wide open mouth and cool air with tightly pursed lips to activate your lover's sensitive thermo-receptors.

Dirty Talk

"Communication outside of the bedroom isn't the only form of dialogue that lays the groundwork for a hot sex life. Research shows that talking about sex during sex leads to higher levels of sexual satisfaction. A study conducted by researchers at Cleveland State University in Ohio found that those who communicate during sex have higher levels of sexual self-esteem and satisfaction. But if dirty talk still isn't on your sexual radar, the same study found that nonverbal communication cues also boost sexual enjoyment."
— From Sex Geeks

Dirty talk is the skill that all good lovers have in common. Once you learn to talk your lover's ear off in bed, you'll barely need to move a muscle— other than your tongue, of course. This is because dirty talk allows you to bring his hottest fantasies to life in words. Through dirty talk, your nasty little tongue becomes the conduit that bridges his deepest desires with in-the-flesh sex. And since fantasy is almost always hotter than reality, fulfilling his desires through dirty talk can be hotter than the real thing. So get ready to whisper sweet (or not-so-sweet) nothings in his ear and watch the fireworks unfold!

Many people find dirty talk off-putting or embarrassing because they derive their definitions and expectations from porn. This leaves them with a terribly limited repertoire that often excludes the highly personal element of individual fantasy. The content of mainstream porn also suggests that all dirty talk must be raunchy, hard core, and deeply rooted in gendered stereotypes of sexual experience. In reality, nothing could be further from the truth.

Dirty talk does not need to be rough, naughty, or even sexual to be erotic. The most enticing chatter can be romantic, teasing, alluring, and flirtatious according to your personal preferences. If you're new to talking dirty, begin with some generous but honest verbal feedback that includes moans, groans, deep exhales, or other sounds to let your lover know that you're enjoying yourself. Don't feel the need to exaggerate—sexy talk is even hotter when you let the tension mount gradually.

Start Small

When you're ready, toss in a few words and short phrases ranging from "Yes!," *"More!,"* and *"Ahhh"* to *"Whoa!," "Wow,"* and *"Fuck yeah!"*

Use language that comes naturally to you, as opposed to repeating what you have seen in films or read online. And since dirty talk goes both ways, use a few simple lines to develop greater comfort as you explore your lover's body: *"Do you like that?" "Where do you want it?" "What can I do for you?" "Tell me how you like it." "Lie back and let me give it to you."*

Indulge Your Sense of Humor

As you integrate dirty talk into your sexual repertoire, remember that it is okay to giggle a little. Obviously you don't want to laugh at your lover, but having a healthy sense of humor will help to ease the tension when you are experimenting with new language, tone, and subject matter. In fact, using a bit of humor and playfulness may be the ideal approach if talking dirty makes you blush or if you're worried about how your lover will respond.

Set Ground Rules

If you are going to continue to expand your dirty talk repertoire, chat with your partner ahead of time about topics, fantasies, or words that are off-limits. Each person has her own unique set of limitations and sensitivities. Maybe your partner likes to use the word pussy, but it makes you angry—not a good mood to be in in the sack! Since these sensitivities can change over time, it's a good idea to revisit your ground rules periodically.

Remember that sex talk isn't enjoyable to all people, especially those who have survived a sexual hardship. **As Dr. Ruth Neustifter (aka Dr.Ruthie) notes**, *"The purpose of talking dirty is to help you both feel excited and intimate, not to feel awkward or triggered! Explicit language can be fun, but it's not erotic for everyone and that'sokay."*

Experiment with Variety

Dirty talk comes in many forms, so experiment with a variety of styles to find the ones that suit you both best. Whether you prefer to be romantic, alluring, teasing, aggressive, demanding, responsive, descriptive, naughty, instructive, ego-stroking, or fantastical is entirely up to you!

Play with these lines on your own in front of the mirror or while masturbating as you get comfortable with your own personal style:

Romantic
"You're the only one for me!"

"I'll only ever want you."

"You're everything I've ever dreamed of."

"You're my dream guy/girl."

Alluring

"I know you want what's under this shirt."

"Tell me what you'd do to me."

"Make my thighs wet!"

"I'll do whatever you tell me to do."

Teasing

"You can't have me."

"If you want it, come and get it."

"Pour me a glass of wine and I'll think about it . . ."

"You know you want it."

Aggressive

"I'm going to hold you down and make you come."

"Behave or I'll give you something to scream about."

"Do as you're told if you want a piece of me."

"Take it!"

Demanding

"Lay me down and take care of me now!"

"Get down on your knees and do it how I like it."

"I want it in my mouth."

"Suck it."

Responsive

"Tell me how you like it."
"What can I do for you?"
"I'm just going to lie back and let you work me over."
"It feels so good."

Desciptive

"I'm going to make you scream."
"I'm coming!"
"I can see your hot body in the mirror."
"It feels so good."

Naughty

"I want to taste your hot cum."
"I thought about you last night when I was touching myself."
"Tie me down and have your way with me."
"I want to be your hot slut."

Instructive

"Put your hand right here!"
"Nibble on me a little."
"Don't stop!"
"Put in your mouth."

Ego-Stroking

"You're the best I've ever had."
"You make me so wet/horny/excited."
"You taste like honey."

"I would pay for this!"

Fantastical
"I want to watch you with another man."
"Let's have a little threesome and let her taste your big cock."
"I want to be tied up and spanked until I can't take it anymore."
"Tie me down and force it down my throat."

Tender Kisses

One of the surest ways you can tell if you want to go further with a partner is to test the waters with kissing. If a man or a woman is too eager, and rushes past the subtle and whispery beginnings, you need to slow the pace. Immediate hard and wet mouth mauling misses the point. Discovery by tongue is a tender, playful journey.

Start out slowly and leisurely with your kissing. How lightly can you kiss? With a relaxed, soft mouth, graze over his cheeks and facial features by barely touching the skin. Trace the eyebrows with soft lips. Tenderly kiss the tip of his nose and the corners of his lips. The mouth, not your hand, becomes the sensatefocus tool.

Breathe lightly into an ear and lick its contour. The mouth is so sensitive that less is often more. Your lips and tongue are exploring and discovering each nook and mound. Your attitude is inquisitive—playing a new game with each kiss. Once you reach his mouth, kiss lightly without your tongue at first.

Special Kisses. For variety, try some fruity kisses. Blindfold your partner and have slices of fresh fruit to share with him when you are the active one in the kissing game. Rub his lips with pineapple, running the cool, textured sweetness over his lips. Lick the juice off his lips. Tease a raspberry onto his tongue. Loll it gently around with your tongue. Bite into a slice of mango and feather it into his mouth. Share in the juices. Switch roles.

The Soft-Lipped Kiss. Some people believe that the world is divided into two types of kissers: soft-lipped and firmlipped. But the reality is that our sexual style varies according to our mood just as our appetite changes from day to day. If your lover seeks romance and often needs help relaxing to get in the mood, slide your lips gently against his with only featherlight contact. Take your time and gently pucker his lower lip between your lips, allowing your easy breathing to slow his breath rate and send his body into a state of deep relaxation.

Lip Lining. Give your honey a peek into your oral skills as you masterfully trace your tongue around the curves of her lips, paying extra attention to the thin skin in the corners where the upper and lower lips meet. If her lips remain closed, sensually slide your tongue from one side to the other just inside the crease.

Sweet Spot. You're probably familiar with the frenulum of the penis, but this sensitive connective tissue also exists just inside the lips. Slide your tongue inside and twirl it purposefully around the shallow space between his upper lips and teeth before moving on to deep, French kissing.

Basic Tongue Twirl. As you press your lips together, tilt your head slightly to the side and suck gently as you twirl your tongue around hers.

Top-Shelf Kiss. Swipe your tongue along the roof of your lover's mouth, a sensitive and oft-neglected area.

Code Word. Kiss your lover out in public at every stoplight, or come up with a code word (e.g., thank you or fun) and stop what you're doing to French kiss whenever you hear this buzzword.

Facial. Hold one another by the cheeks as you kiss deeply and passionately. The face is the most sensual part of the body but receives little attention in the way of touch.

The Rocket

The Rocket is one of the most versatile finger and tongue tricks designed to make her toes curl at any stage of the sexual response cycle. Whether you want to seduce her into your arms or bring her to the heights of an earth-shattering orgasm, this will become a go-to move for years to come.

Take Position

You can use the Rocket technique in almost any position. Whether you're sitting side-by-side at dinner or lying on the couch watching a movie, as long as you can cup her mons into your hand and reach your fingers down against her lips, you're ready to go!

The Moves

■ Place your palm flat against her mons and bend your fingers down to press against the full width and length of her vulva so that you're cupping it in your hand.

■ Slowly slide your fingers up and down ever so slightly, maintaining pressure against her mons and clitoris.

■ If you're able, continue to slide your fingers up and down as you slip your tongue between the grooves of your fingers to tease her inner lips.

■ Increase the pressure and speed of your fingers, paying special attention to the very top of her vulva as she becomes more aroused.

Sit On My Face

This oral sex move allows her to maintain complete control as she directs the pressure, depth, speed, and motion with her hips. Her directives not only ensure that she gets it exactly as she pleases, but her dominance offers great practice in sexual assertion.

If you love the Sit on My Face technique but want to keep things fresh, simply change directions to face his feet and ask him to finger your bum a little at the same time.

Take Position

Lie on your back and prop your head up with a few pillows. Have her kneel over your lower face with her back to your feet so that you can use eye contact as a means of communicating while your mouth is full.

The Moves

How she sits on your face is entirely up to her, but here are a few suggestions for her:

■ Rock your hips back and forth in an elliptical fashion.

■ Demand that he stick his tongue straight up as you pop up and down over it.

■ Apply some lube and slide back and forth over the full length of his face.

■ Rub your wet pussy against his chin and closed lips with firm pressure.

■ Sway your hips from side to side in a semi-circle.

■ Sit hard on his mouth and instruct him to suck away.

■ Ask him to stick his tongue out flat against his chin and grind up on it.

TIP: Slide three wet fingers beneath your mouth and stroke her sweet spot (perineum) from back to front in rhythm with your tongue twirling.

Suck and Seal

This technique not only combines licking, sucking, and deep pressure, but it also provides full-contact stimulation of the entire vulva.

By wrapping your mouth all the way around the outer edges of her pussy, you'll titillate and awaken all the inner and outer components of her highly responsive clitoris.

Take Position

Kneel on a pillow on the floor next to the bed as she lies down with her knees bent and legs hanging off the edge.

The Moves

■ Tease all around her pussy with some gentle breath kisses without allowing your lips to contact her skin. Breathe heavily over her thighs and mons, allowing your cheeks and nose to touch her only incidentally.

■ With a wide, flat tongue lick from the very bottom of her vulva up to the top as slowly as possible. Repeat this lick in the same direction for thirty to sixty seconds.

■ Switch directions and lick from her clitoral glans down to her fourchette (where her inner labia meet at the bottom) using the warm, flat underside of your tongue. Repeat for another minute.

■ When she starts to thrust her hips into you, open your mouth wide and press your lips around the outer edges of her vulva.

■ Sweep your tongue around the inside perimeter of your lips while sucking and slurping away.

The Lollipops

If you want to spread her orgasmic sensations across the entire surface of her pussy and beyond, then the Lollipops move is right up your alley. Using sweeping motions to stroke the bulbs of her inner clitoris from the top of her clitoral glans to her fourchette down below, this move provides the intense stimulation most women require to reach the heights of sexual pleasure.

Take Position

Kneel between her legs as she sits (or lies) atop a table with her legs hanging off the edge.

The Moves

■ Warm her up with a gentle thigh massage by circling with only the palms of your hands slathered in coconut oil.

■ As her body begins to relax into your hands, slide one palm up to her mons and press down gently as the other flat palm circles slowly around her entire vulva.

■ Lick her pussy like a lollipop with a soft flat tongue, starting from the fourchette at the very bottom all the way up to the clitoral glans at the top. Alternate from the "left lane" of her vulva to the "right lane" as you separate her lips with your tongue with each stroke.

■ Between each lick, wrap your lips around the tiny fourchette at the base as you suck gently. Then press your tongue firmly into her clit at the top

TIPS: *Twirl your tongue around her fourchette and then lick with a wide, flat tongue up to her clit before encircling it with the tip of your tongue.*

Stroking the Shaft

For many women, the shaft of the clitoris offers an immense sense of pleasure, and, just like men, orgasm is often the result of a rhythmic stroking motion.

Slide your smooth fingers over this hot spot while simultaneously kissing and rubbing her inner clitoral legs and bulbs to send her into sensory overload.

Take Position

Prop up her hips and lower back with at least two pillows and spread her legs wide as she bends her knees. Slide between her open legs and dive on in!

The Moves

■ Press your full lips against her vulva and slide them up and down.

■ Move your entire head in a circular fashion to encircle her entire pussy with your wet lips.

■ Pulse your lips against her as you slide your tongue inside and curl it up against her soft, inner walls.

■ Add your fingers into the mix according to your preferences as you increase the pace, depth, and intensity of your tongue screw

■ As her arousal levels rise, press your tongue flat against her vulva and stroke from side to side.

■ Continue to shake your head from side to side with your tongue pressed into her and place one thumb on her clitoral hood. Draw her skin up and down with your thumb to stroke the shaft and produce a climactic finale.

TIPS: *Stroke the shaft from behind by having her lie on her stomach and sliding a hand beneath the lower part of her pubic mound. She can use her body weight to grind away as you lick, kiss, and suck her pussy from behind.*

G-spot Gusher

Get her wet and let her gush as you excite her G-spot from all angles and leave her dripping at the thighs. Alternate the "come hither" motion against her G-spot with some deep circular pressure. Draw circles or ovals on the upper vaginal wall, against the G-spot. You should feel the area swell as circulation and arousal rise.

Remember that the G-spot isn't a distinct organ but an area of the body that is associated with the release of fluids. Each woman's experience with the G-spot is unique, and the degree of pleasure associated with this sensitive area can vary according to a number of factors, including arousal levels and monthly cycle.

Take Position

Kneel at her feet as she stands with her back against a wall.

The Moves

■ Play with your surefire warm-up moves that you know she loves before moving on to her sensitive G-spot.

■ Once she's all fired up and ready to go, slide your index and middle fingers inside of her and curl them up against the front wall of her vagina (toward her stomach).

■ Curl them in a "come hither" motion, gradually increasing the pressure and speed, up to at least two "curls" per second. As you curl your fingers inside of her, wrap your lips around the glans of her clit and pulse in tempo with your fingers.

■ Finally, press your lower palm down against her lower abdomen to squeeze and excite her prostate from the inside-out.

TIP: *Though squirting isn't a sideshow trick, and not every woman will experience the same degree of ejaculation, you can encourage fluid expulsion by bearing down with your pelvic floor muscles. As you approach orgasm, take a few deep breaths as you "push out" with the muscles around your vagina.*

Tongue Screw

As your nimble fingers press into her G-spot and squeeze her clitoris, your tongue works its magic against her responsive lower wall, resulting in a climactic flurry of nerve-ending responses.

Take Position

Kneel behind her as she lies flat on her stomach with her legs hanging off the bed and her feet on the floor. Approaching from behind will facilitate the dual entry of your fingers in alignment with your tongue.

The Moves

■ Sweep your fingers gently over her butt cheeks and tease her perineum as you breathe over her pussy from behind. With your palm facing downward, slide your index finger inside of her and slip your thumb beneath her.

■ Gently pinch your thumb and index finger together so that your thumb presses against her clit and your index finger curls against her G-spot along the front wall.

■ Angle your other knuckles downward to make space for your tongue. Slide your tongue inside of her against your index finger and curl upward (toward the back wall of her vagina) as you continue the pinching motion.

Slippery Palm

The Slippery Palm technique puts you in the driver's seat as you use your strong hands to hold her open and leave her feeling vulnerable to your sexual prowess. Her most sensitive areas will be exposed, so encourage her to embrace the submissive role as you work your magic between her legs.

Take Position

Sweep her off of her feet and place her on the bed. Reassure her that she's in good hands. Lie on a pillow between her legs as she rests her feet (legs bent) on your shoulders. Place a few pillows under her hips for easy access as she lies on her back.

The Moves

■ Tie a blindfold loosely around her eyes.

■ S-l-o-w-l-y kiss your way down from her neck to her inner thighs, stopping to show some love to her collarbone, nipples, underarms, hips bones, and bellybutton along the way.

■ Slip both palms in between her legs and warm up her thighs with soft, circular strokes as you kiss her mons with wet lips and a swirling tongue.

■ Press your palms into her vulva and use your thumbs to separate her inner lips and reveal the shiny space between them.

■ Sweep your tongue around this opening while you press your thumbs gently against her inner lips and slide them ever-so-slightly up and down.

■ Use the textured upper side of your tongue to trace a large X over her exposed area and moan a little to let her know you're enjoying yourself.

■ If she seems tense or tries to close her legs at all, scold her gently: "You're all mine and I'm going to take care of you, so you best behave."

■ Open your mouth wide and press your lips and flat tongue against her vestibule as you slide from top to bottom while sucking away.

TIPS: *Practice this one on your finger to familiarize yourself with the sensation of suction created by a cradled tongue. You should almost be able to hold your finger in place with the sides of your tongue as they curl up around your finger.*

Slow Thrust

A common mistake that a lot of men make when it comes to sex is going too far too fast. One of the things that women love during sex is teasing and anticipation. Women can go absolutely crazy if you show them something they want, but don't give it them straight away. Most men do the complete opposite when it comes to sex. As soon as they get their penis in their woman they put it in all the way and start thrusting super fast. What does this leave the woman to look forward to and anticipate? Nothing. And often this kills all the sexual tension and makes you as the guy have to work 10 times as hard to get her to orgasm. Many times women will love it if you start sex very slowly with foreplay.

Take Position

Sweep her off of her feet and place her on the bed. Reassure her that she's in good hands.

The Moves

■ Start by entering your penis inside her very slowly by only half an inch and then pulling it out.

■ Then next time put it in very slowly three quarters of an inch and then pull it out. Then keep thrusting slowly in and out at that depth for a bit.

■ A minute or so later thrust just a little bit deeper.

■ Try moving your hips in circles instead of just back and forth. This can offer some grinding stimulation for your clit.

■ And aim for it to be roughly 5 minutes into having sex before you're actually thrusting at full depth.

Hitting G-spot

When you massage the Grafenberg spot with your penis during intercourse you have to remember to aim for the spot. Most men will just get lost in the pleasure of thrusting, but it is necessary to thrust in the right area to produce fantastic results. Some positions will make your target much easier to hit than others. One of the easiest positions to do this successfully with is missionary.

Traditional missionary will work just fine, however a man has to be very hard to have his penis arch up slightly to massage the spongy area that is about two inches inside the top of the vaginal canal. You want to do off the bed missionary, which entails having your lover waist at the edge of the bed.

Take Position

Her legs will be dangling over the edge, while her back and head while be on the bed.

The Moves

■ You should come into her from an upward angle and have her legs wrapped gently around your thighs.

■ This allows you to thrust up into the spot and drive her wild.

■ Remember that the area is not that deep. So what you need to do is slide the head of your penis down the top of her vaginal canal.

■   Start from the very beginning of the vaginal opening and use almost a thrust glide. This will have her in complete erotic bliss.

Missionary drive

I believe that you know what is missionary position. The Missionary style is the basic and most used position during sexual intercourse. Have your partner lie down flat on her back and her legs open. You then position yourself on top of her while she wraps her legs around your waist, holding you tight against her.

The Missionary is great as it allows intimacy between the two of you, as both you and your partner can look each other in the eyes and kiss at the same time while achieve deep penetration. This will make your partner feel a great sense of closeness and bring her to a mind blowing orgasm.

Take Position

Now, change from normal style, you let her spread her leg wide open, either resting on your chest or hanging freely in the air, she is lying on the bed. You should knee down in between her widely opened legs and give her the thrust that will eventually make her drop into heavy orgasm.

The Moves

- First, you should start to thrust slowly and stimulate her interest by giving her some rub and caress on her breast and other sensitive body parts, let her feel the sexual tension and excitement.

- If her reaction is good, gradually increase the thrust speed and give her deeper penetration.

- Play with her clitoris if necessary.

- Kiss her when you are in action, the pressure you put on her when you lean forward will grant you a deeper penetration and give her more sexual arousal!

Chapter 4: Steps to a Better Sex Life

What to do Before Sex

Nutrition

In order to have better sex it is necessary to keep the penis and reproductive organs in a healthy state. For optimum performance and for increased libido, it is vital to keep the arteries healthy in order to allow increased blood flow to the penis.

The Role of Testosterone in Male Sexual Health

Testosterone is the prominent male sex hormone produced by the testicles and adrenal glands, and is crucial in the development of male characteristics of genital sexual progression. Testosterone is vital in the functions of penis growth, muscle development, sperm production, and sex drive in regards to genital sexual health. In order to increase libido and counter erectile dysfunction it is necessary to increase testosterone levels.

A poor diet can lead to a lackluster sex life, while some foods have the power to make you last longer in bed. A healthy balance of vitamins and minerals keeps your endocrine system humming, which in turn regulates the production of the hormones estrogen and testosterone, essential for sexual desire and performance, says *Cammi Balleck, PhD, a naturopathic physician and author of Making Happy Happen. "Enjoying an active sex life is essential to our wellbeing, and the foods we eat play a large role in ensuring we feel in the mood," she says.* So you could call good food and good sex a positive feedback loop.

Here are foods with proven power to make you last longer:

Lobster

Sure, part of its appeal is the special-occasion nature, not to mention all that licking of butter off your fingers. But you may eschew this crustacean in fear that a heavy, fatty meal will slow you down sexually.

Turns out, lobster doesn't deserve its tag as a high-fat food (except when slathered in said butter!). In fact, it's a good source of lean protein, copper, zinc and selenium. Zinc, in particular, has been linked with a healthy male libido.

Lobster is also chock full of the mineral phosphorus, which boosts both your sex drives. Plus, its concentration of essential fatty acids may increase sensitivity in your sex organs.

Leafy Green Veggies

It may not be easy being green, but it is sexy. Kale, spinach and other leafy greens are high in vitamin A, which is a great hormone-balancer because it supports proper endocrine function. These foods also contain iodine, an essential mineral for proper function of your thyroid and adrenal glands, which in turn help regulate your mood. It's hard to feel great about sex if you don't feel, well, great, so fill up on some greens.

Strawberries

It's not just that these sweet, juicy fruits look and feel sexy (heck, they wear their fertility —their seeds—on the outside!). The health benefits that they pack give weight to their aphrodisiacal reputation. Aside from a ridiculously high amount of vitamin C, folic acid and fiber, strawberries are a good source of potassium, which helps you avoid fluid retention. They even contain omega-3 fatty acids, highly valued for their contribution to a healthy cardiovascular system. And that's essential for sexual arousal and responsiveness.

Dark Chocolate

Put aside for a moment how good it tastes and feels as it melts in your mouth—which is enough proof for most chocolate lovers that chocolate is for lovers. Dark chocolate contains a compound called phenylethylamine, an endorphin released in the brain when you're feeling the warm fuzzies of falling in love. Share a few squares of high-quality dark chocolate before bed, and hopping in the sack will feel all the more delicious.

Nuts

Many varieties, including walnuts, hazelnuts, almonds, pine nuts, Brazil nuts and peanuts, contain the essential amino acid l-arginine, which helps the brain do its job circulating neurotransmitters, brain chemicals that send messages to cells (like, "gee, this feels so good—more please!").

And the fatty acids in nuts increase endorphins, making you feel more relaxed. L-arginine also has been shown to dilate blood vessels, improving blood flow to the genitals, which in turn may enhance arousal and intensify orgasms.

Blueberries

Circulation is a big deal for both libido and sexual function—without good blood flow, arousal takes longer (it's the blood rushing to your sexy bits that primes you for orgasm)—and blueberries are great for improving circulation.

Their high levels of antioxidants, which destroy cell-damaging free radicals, also make you look sexier. What's more: Blueberries contain dopamine, a neurotransmitter whose job is to stimulate your brain's pleasure centers (the ones that make you say, "Ooh!").

Watermelon

True, cool and juicy slabs of watermelon are a staple at G-rated family picnics, but this super-sweet fruit is also asex-booster. First, bright-red watermelon contains an amino acid called l-citrulline, which helps relax and dilate blood vessels, naturally increasing blood flow to sexual organs and contributing to a hotter climax. Plus, watermelon's mostly, you know, water—making it an anti-bloat machine. Incorporating a pit-spitting contest into sex play: Optional.

Asparagus

Asparagus is rich in vitamin B6 and folate, both of which can boost arousal and orgasm. It also boasts vitamin E, which stimulates sex hormones in men and women.

Avocado

Energy and libido are crucial for sex, and avocados can give you both. They're loaded with minerals, monounsaturated fats (the good kind that protect the heart and lower cholesterol), and vitamin B6 – all of which help keep your energy and sex drive up. They're also a top source of omega-3 fatty acids, which naturally boost your mood.

Chile Peppers

Chile peppers can really spice things up thanks to capsaicin, a chemical that's been shown to induce the release of endorphins in the brain, which create a feeling of euphoria.

Seafood

Seafood is a real source of having a good blood flow. With a smooth blood flow a man would never feel tired and would never have to deal with low sex drive. Seafood can do the magic of performing better in bed.

Onion

Onion soup also comes in the list for foods for sex as it can digest the food quickly hence leaving a man feeling light and in a better mood to have sex rather than being in an annoyed state of mind.

Almonds

Almonds are rich in potassium and vitamin E and they help in increasing the stamina of sex in men that eventually helps them perform better in bed.

Eggs

Egg boosts your sex drive naturally. Daily intake 2 to 3 eggs will increases testosterone levels and also benefits for premature ejaculation

Carrots

Carrots are filled with vitamins and minerals. Carrots help to strengthen penile muscles as well and help in regulating blood flow to the male sex organ

Oats

Oats helps reducing anxiety and stress. Premature ejaculation linked with stress and anxiety Banana

Physical Exercises

If you cannot start exercising for the sake of your fitness and health, maybe the possibility of improving your sex life might drive you to taking it a little more seriously. Exercise will not only make you look better, which definitely makes it easier to attract the opposite sex, but it can also enhance your ability and performance and make it a lot more fun. There is a direct relationship between a lack of physical exercise and sex, which many medical studies have proven, therefore, if you do not want to be remembered for being a miserable partner, I suggest that you start taking your health and fitness a little more seriously and understand the difference it can make in your sex life.

Here are top eight exercises:

Pushups

If you're going to pick just one exercise to do, this is the one to go for. For all the obvious reasons. If you can't do basic training, quality pushups at first, start with wall presses (essentially pushups done against the wall), aiming for 3 sets of 12 to 15 repetitions.

When you're ready, progress to knee pushups on the floor, making sure to keep your back straight (squeeze your butt and suck in your gut) while you slowly touch your nose to the ground. Once you're ready to kick it up a notch, progress to traditional hand and toe pushups.

Crunches

Your abs are a critical sex boosting body area to work on. After all, you have to use your abdominal muscles during sex. Starting your ab workout with good old fashioned crunches. Lie on your back, hands supporting your neck, knees bent, and your feet on the floor. Then bring your body up just enough to get your shoulders off the ground. Do 3 to 5 sets of 15 to 20 repetitions.

Bridges

Men and women also do bridges. Lying on your back, knees bent, feet on the floor, lift your hips up and down for 3 sets of 15 reps. You can also try pelvic tilts. Standing up or lying down, straighten your lower back and pull your belly button in until your lower back touches the wall or floor.

Deadlifts

This exercise will keep your back as strong as it can be, and give your legs and torso a workout too. Deadlifts, in which you start in a neutral bent-over position and raise a weighted barbell or dumbbells from the ground, are easy to do and easy to do wrong. So technique is important to prevent injury. Get some pro tips online or at your gym to be sure you're getting the most out of doing deadlifts

Torso side bends and twists

To get the most from this exercise, as well as the next one, head to the gym. The effort is worth it because torso side bends and twists will keep your upper body strong, and give you stamina. Do them on the cable crossover machine for maximum effect. Pushing or pulling exercise in the gym. Rows, flyes, and lateral raises on the cable crossover machine will do a great job of enhancing your performance in the bedroom. Remember to get a few quick tips from a pro on how to do these exercises most effectively.

Yoga

Yoga strengthens your pelvic muscles and increases your sexual flexibility and energy. Poses such as the elbow balance, shoulder stand, and bow pose can enhance your pelvic muscles, while triangle pose, pigeon, and standing forward bend can improve flexibility.

One of the more recently published studies of the impact of yoga on male sexual function involved 65 men ages 24 to 60. After 12 weeks of yoga sessions, "male sexual quotient" scores significantly improved in the areas of orgasm, ejaculatory control, erection, confidence, intercourse satisfaction, sexual desire, and performance. Basically what that means is that all these guys doing yoga in the test had better sex because of their yoga practice.

Kegel Exercises

Kegels are a sexercise you can do just about anywhere, anytime without breaking a sweat, and without anyone actually knowing you are doing them. Kegels are usually thought of as an exercise for just women, but they are equally beneficial for men's sexual health.

If you have ever consciously stopped your flow of urine for several seconds when going to the bathroom, then you have exercised your pubococcygeus (PC) muscles. I've found that practicing this squeezing action several times a day (hold the squeeze for 10 seconds, relax, and repeat 8 or more times), can strengthen your pelvic floor muscles, which in turn can help you delay ejaculation, have better control over your orgasm, and experience better sex.

Stretching

I've found that certain stretches like "pelvic stretching" can enhance your orgasms and keep you flexible and injury-free while having sex.

Here's how you do them: Wearing comfortable clothes, lie on your back on the floor on a mat. Bend your knees and place your feet on the floor slightly apart. Place your arms at your sides. Inhale and simultaneously tighten your abdominals and buttocks while lifting your pelvis until your back is straight. Hold this position for 10 seconds or more, then exhale and lower your body. Repeat several times.

Set yourself a calendar reminder to do them first thing in the morning. Trust me – they work. If you don't adopt any of the other recommendations in this section, do this one!

Great sex has many components — physical, emotional, nutritional, and psychological. Exercise is the best way to maintain your physical health, which also goes a long way toward having better sex and stronger erectile function for men.

What to do During Sex

Using Condoms

One method that has that has become very popular as a technique to prevent premature ejaculation is condom usage.

Many times I have heard men and women often complain of the desensitizing tendencies of a condom. Many couples despised using the rubber because they said they could not completely feel the pleasure of doing intercourse with it. But, fortunately for those with premature ejaculation problems, this is a great (not to mention cheap) way of addressing your premature ejaculation. It may not be a completely justified premature ejaculation treatment in itself but it may help when used in a full blown premature ejaculation treatment.

Men who have problems with penile hypersensitivity may find it difficult to employ the breathing technique successfully. That 's because regardless of how much control they have over their breathing, they still wouldn't be able to control the onslaught of sensation on the penile nerves. In this case, the best option is to pair up the technique with delay condoms.

Gone are the days when condoms only served one purpose: to avoid conception. Nowadays, there seems to be a condom that promises to address every conceivable sexual problem on the planet including premature ejaculation. Delay condoms are relatively new and were specifically designed to help men last longer than normal during intercourse. Men who can last for more than a minute after penetration no longer need to use delay condoms. That ' s because regular condoms can often efficiently do the job of delaying ejaculation.

But men with hypersensitive penises need the help delay condoms because their penises often remain sensitive despite the coverage of a regular condom. There are different types of delay condoms that these men can choose from, namely:

Delay condoms that are thicker than normal condoms. These condoms work like any other normal condoms except that the thickness ensures that the man feels less friction during penetration. The numbing effect is almost immediate as soon as the condom wraps around the penis. This means that the couple can go on with the intercourse right away.

Delay condoms that contain either one of two numbing agents that are often used as local anesthetics: benzocaine or lidocaine. The chemical is contained within the condom ' s inner body. It normally takes up to 2 minutes after the penis comes into contact with the chemical before the numbing effect fully sets in.

This means that men would have to put on the condom before starting foreplay. Another option is to find creative ways of delaying penetration while waiting for their penises to numb.

Men who opt for delay condoms that contain numbing agents have to be very careful, though. That ' s because the numbing agent is so effective that it can also cause their partners ' sexual organs to grow numb as well if it ever comes into contact with the chemicals. The chemicals may also cause allergic reactions if either the man or his partner ' s sexual organ is sensitive to its components.

Some men might want to try applying benzocaine or lidocaine directly on their penises without the use of a condom. This is a big no-no for the reason stated above: the numbing agent can also numb their partners ' nerves. This can result in a really uncomfortable and often painful sexual session.

However if you want to use regular condoms, you can apply the following tips to avoid quick ejaculation:

■ **First of all DO NOT get the "ultra thin" brands of condoms.** This is the opposite of what we are trying to achieve. We don't want things to be more sensitive! This will just encourage quick ejaculation. So avoid these brands even though they are pushed heavily and advertised as if they are one's to go with.

■ **Double Up.** This is a trick not many guys have figured out, but it actually works pretty good. Instead of slipping on one condom, slip on two. This greatly decreases the intense sensations which cause us to ejaculate too quickly. A second condom can add several minutes to your lasting ability.

■ **Cream Condoms.** There are some condoms out there which actually contain cream inside them that will numb up your penis somewhat so that you don't get over excited and feel the intense stimulations during sex. Now this can be a hit or miss, as some guys can get so numbed that they don't feel a whole lot of anything. But if you are extremely sensitive then this option can work very well for you as it will allow much longer lasting time than usual.

These are all good methods that can be used immediately. The best strategy is to use these methods while you are learning the exercises and techniques we will discuss in next chapter. That way you can still have sex while at the same time you are working towards naturally improving your lasting power permanently.

Remember that when doing sexual activity with a condom, the female partner's vaginal canal must be fully lubricated. Otherwise, it might be hard for the penis to penetrate the vagina without much lubrication. Having said that, proper foreplay and oral or manual stimulation must be done minutes before the planned penetration begins.

Control Your Breathing

In this section, we are going to talk the importance of breathing in order to stay in control of your arousal and a specific breathing technique that make will you last longer in bed.

You see, If you can control your breath, you can control your body. If you were looking for a magic pill that solves all problems with no efforts on your part, well I'm sorry to tell you that such thing doesn't exist. Like anything of value in life, learning how to make love for longer requires some work. But breathing really is the closest thing to a magic pill.

The breath is the link between what you can't control and what you can control in your body. For example, you can't control your heart, you can't tell your heart to stop beating. On the other hand, you can fully control the movements of your arms or your hands. Breathing is somewhere in the middle.

If you don't think about breathing, you breath anyway, and that's obviously a good thing – we don't have to always think about breathing in order to survive! But you can also control your breathing, focus on it and modify it in order to change what's happening in your body. With your breathing, you can control stress and fear, and you can also control your sexual arousal and last longer during sex.

Simply using deep breathing and focusing on your breathing will allow you to decrease your arousal level significantly in no time, and at will. When I say *"deep breathing"*, I mean a breath that starts from the belly. Don't breathe from your chest; it has to start from your belly.

Breathing Techniques To Increase bedroom Stamina

■ Now, I want you to simply start putting all your attention on your breathing. Focus on your inhalations and your exhalations. Notice how only focusing on it makes you breathe more slowly and deeply. Notice how you already feel more relaxed, more in control of what's happening in your body.

■ Now, try a few deep breaths. Again, I want you to focus only on your breathing. Visualize the air first filling your belly, then rising to your rib cage, then to your heart and then to your throat; be aware of those 4 points as you inhale.

■ When you exhale, just let go of all the air and relax. Don't force the air out of your lungs but just let go. Don't be shy – you can even make a little sound like "haaaaaaa" as you release the air.

OK, so now that you know that breathing is one of the keys to control your climax, and now that you know what deep breathing is, you can incorporate it in your practice. When you masturbate , be focused on your body and your sensations. Also, be aware of your arousal and where you are on a scale of 1 to 10; it shouldn't be too hard to focus on your breathing at the same time.

Whenever you feel your arousal going up faster than you would like, focus on your breathing and start doing deep breaths as I just described.

I can guarantee that this alone will bring your arousal back down and give you more control. And by the way, you can do the same during intercourse. There's nothing wrong with focusing on your breathing or using deep breathing while making love.

It will definitely help you last longer and your partner might even find it sexy. (Especially when she realizes you're in control and you're present in the moment!) But if you're worried that she might think you're doing something weird, why don't you share with her what you're trying to accomplish? She can be a great support for you, particularly when she realizes your objective is to make sex better for both of you!

Special Medication

Let's take a quick look at some of the available medications that have potential for improving premature ejaculation. Again, the U.S. Food and Drug Administration hasn't approved any drugs to treat premature ejaculation in particular. All of the options below are prescribed "off label" by physicians, which means that the medication is typically used to treat an-other condition (depression, for example) but shows promise for treating other problems (in this case, premature ejaculation). While these drugs can have side effects, they are generally safe and somewhat effective, and doctors are often willing to prescribe them for premature ejaculation.

Paxil (paroxetine)

■ *Type: SSRI*

■ *Typical dose: 20 mg/day*

■ *Side effects: Nausea, headache, sleepiness, dry mouth, dizziness*

■ *What to Expect: May take 3 to 6 weeks to see benefits for PE; must be taken every day. Should be used with caution by men with liver or kidney disease, bipolar disorder, bleeding disorders, or glaucoma or who have recently had a heart attack*

■ *Notes: May interact with the anti-seizure drug phe-nobarbital, warfarin (Coumadin), alcohol, and some other antidepressants*

Prozac (fluoxetine)

- *Type: SSRI*

- *Typical dose: 10 to 20 mg/day*

- *Side effects: Nausea, headache, insomnia, nervousness, dizziness*

- *What to Expect: May take 3 to 6 weeks to see benefits for PE; must be taken every day. Should be used with caution by men with diabetes or a history of seizures*

- *Notes: May interact with the anti-seizure drug phe-nobarbital, warfarin (Coumadin), lithium, sedatives, alcohol, and some other antidepressants*

Zoloft (sertraline)

- *Type: SSRI*

- *Typical dose: 50 mg/day*

- *Side effects: Nausea, headache, diarrhea, insomnia*

- *What to Expect: May take 3 to 6 weeks to see benefits for PE; must be taken every day. Should be used with caution by men with liver or kidney disease or glaucoma or who have recently had a heart attack*

- *Notes: May interact with warfarin (Coumadin), di-azepam (Valium), sedatives, alcohol, and some other antidepressants*

Priligy (dapoxetine)

- *Type: SSRI*

- *Side effects: Nausea, headache, dizziness, nervousness*

- *What to Expect: Suitable for "on-demand" use—taken before you have sex, not every day*

- *Notes: Not yet available in the U.S. By prescription in some countries, including Germany, Finland, and Sweden*

Viagra

- *Type: Phosphodiesterase type 5 (PDE5) inhibitor*

- *Side effects: Diarrhea, dizziness, facial flushing, stuffy nose, heartburn*

- *Typical dose: Suitable for "on-demand" use—taken before you have sex, not every day. 25 to 50 mg one or two hours before intercourse. Should used with caution by men with high blood pressure or who have recently had a heart attack or stroke. Should not be taken by men who also take nitrates.*

■   *Notes: Interacts with nitrates. May interact with prote-ase inhibitors and some antibiotics*

Chapter 5: Techniques to Fix Premature Ejaculation

Tip 1: Breathing Technique

Breathing exercises focus more on helping men with premature ejaculation address the stress and anxiety that is possibly causing the problem. Experts believe that short, shallow breaths send the wrong signals to the brain, thus triggering the heart to race faster, which then prompts the brain to interpret it as a sign that it ' s time for the brain chemicals to trigger an orgasm.

This is the same principle that is behind the body ' s fight-or-flight response: when the heart is racing fast, the body responds either by fighting or fleeing. In the case of men who suffer from premature ejaculation, the body ' s go-to response is often ' flight ' . This means that it operates under the thought of getting things over with right away so that there ' s still enough time to flee. This response is often attributed with early sexual experiences that may have caused the development of premature ejaculation, specifically the experiences of masturbating discreetly and hurriedly for fear of being caught.

Men with premature ejaculation can regain control of their bodies and its responses to stimuli by simply mastering their breathing. They specifically have to learn how to breathe deeply since deep breathing relaxes the heartbeat. This then signals the brain to hold off the brain chemicals, which in turn delays ejaculation.

The steps for mastering deep breathing to address premature ejaculation are:

■ Sit or lie down in a relaxed position.

■ Perform the same diaphragm breathing that has already been discussed on the previous chapter. Most people unconsciously breathe through the chest instead of the diaphragm. This process often results in shallow breathing that does not help the body relax and has no effects on the blood vessels. It also often causes rapid heart rates that aggravate the symptoms of stress and anxiety. In contrast, breathing through the diaphragm allows men to take deeper breaths. This facilitates the proper flow of oxygen to the lungs and all the other parts of the body including the brain.

■ Hold the breath in for a second and then exhale slowly.

■ Repeat the process for up to 10 repetitions.

Experts suggest that it is best to do this breathing exercise right before sexual intercourse. This gives the body enough time to feel the relaxation that comes as a result of the exercise. It also relieves the brain of the toxic brain chemicals that are associated with stress and anxiety. Doing the breathing exercise during sex is also helpful for men who are anxious about how their partners would rate their sexual performance.

One advantage of consciously doing it during sex is that it allows both partners to regulate their breathing to match each other. Experts believe that this promotes a higher level of intimacy between the couple.

Tip 2: Squeeze Technique

Squeezing is one of the best known exercises used to delay ejaculation. The squeeze technique has been known about for decades. So is it a useful tool that has stood the test of time or are there better methods out there? Find out in this section.

What Is It? This is a method that uses the hands to manipulate the penis and cause it to lose arousal. If you do this repeatedly during sex then you can go for much longer than if you had not used this technique.

What Is The Exact Technique?

This technique can be used both during the sexual act and masturbation.

In this technique, the male is allowed to masturbate so that blood fills up the penis and makes it hard. The masturbation is carried out till a point when the male is just about to discharge the semen. At this point, the glans or the head of the penis, from which the semen is supposed to be discharged, it squeezed so as to prevent the discharge. As a result, the blood flows out of the penis and leaves it flaccid. The process is repeated a number of times in order to increase the time taken for ejaculation to happen. If done successfully, this exercise can very effectively delay ejaculation.

Squeezing needs to be carried out with a lot of care. The masturbation should be done gently to prevent any tearing of the tissue. If the repetition of masturbation makes the male uncomfortable or causes pain in the penis, the exercise should be stopped immediately.

Any Drawbacks?

Some men find it inconvenient to do this technique. Also, you can only practice this technique with a lover that you trust. It is obviously not suitable for women you are having casual sex with or have just met.

Tip 3: Start-Stop Method

This technique can be used both during the sexual act and masturbation. It might be easier to try it out during the masturbation first, so there is no pressure to deal with. This technique requires you to be aware of your body and foresee the point of no return coming up. Point of no return is an instant when the level of arousal suddenly skyrockets and the ejaculation happens several seconds after this moment. Stop and Start technique is performed like this:

■ Start stimulating your penis either through sexual intercourse or masturbation. Stay aware of your body and observe your level of arousal

■   When you feel you are approaching the point of no return, stop all stimulation. The sexual arousal is going to progressively subside.

■   Once your arousal has reached controllable level, you can resume your sexual intercourse or masturbation.

■   Repeat steps 2 and 3 as many times as you wish.

In some cases you do not want your partner to know that you are using this technique to last longer. You might be having a one-night stand; this is when a stealth version of this method comes into play. What you do is as you feel the point of no return approaching, pull out and change positions. This will give you around 10 seconds to reduce your arousal level. If you feel like you need more time, you can also perform some oral sex (this will be discuss later in this chapter) on your partner. This way your partner will receive a great deal of sexual pleasure and will stay clueless of the fact that you are utilizing this technique.

Tip 4: Mutual Masturbation

Mutual masturbation (masturbating with a partner) is a really safe way to have sex and let the other person know what feels good to you. But there's no rule against sharing masturbatory activities with a partner, especially if that partner is willing to join in and masturbate themselves as well. When a guy practices proper penis care, his penis is in very presentable shape and can join in a mutual masturbation session with no worry about how he looks. But changing the solo activity into a duet can take some preparation.

This assumes, of course, that a man is interested in mutual masturbation with his partner in an existing relationship (whether of sexual exclusivity or not). There are some other situations in which a man can masturbate openly with another person (or persons) who are essentially strangers. For example, many masturbation clubs exist, some catering to men only, some to both male and female participants. In such situations, the only preparation required is for the man to locate such a club and find out its meeting places, times and rules.

A partner

But assuming a man is talking about masturbating in tandem with a recognized partner, the situation may require some forethought. Here are some things to consider before asking a partner to join in a stoke- or rub-fest.

■ Has masturbation been mentioned before? In the relationship, have either one of the participants ever brought up the subject, even in a playful way? If so, what was said and what kind of response did it evoke? If it has not been mentioned, is that significant, or is it merely that the subject never arose?

■ What kind of sexual views does the partner have? Sometimes (although not always) a guy can make a pretty good guess about how his partner feels about masturbation based on their embracing or rejecting of other sexual matters. For example, a partner who rips their clothes off when sex is proposed and jumps on the bed growling may be more open to the idea of mutual masturbation than a partner who insists on turning all the lights off before disrobing.

■ How touchy-feely is the partner where genitals are concerned? Is sex typically all about penetration (or perhaps all about oral sex), or do the participants already fondle each other's genitals in the course of their lovemaking?

Assuming the answers to these questions indicate a likely willingness or interest in a masturbation duet, the man may want to move forward - although still with caution if he is unsure of how the partner might respond.

Each couple is different, so there is no hard and fast rule as to whether to approach the subject jokingly, seriously, playfully, etc. Whatever approach is made, a guy should be prepared for some negative reactions.

For example, a partner may find the idea distasteful. If so, this will hopefully be expressed in a sensitive manner. Similarly, some partners may mistakenly believe a guy is suggesting this approach because he doesn't find the couple's current sexual activities satisfying. The man should firmly reassure the partner that this is not the case and that he is simply looking to explore new ways of sharing their sexual selves.

Tip 5: Relaxation Techniques

The following exercise will teach you how to relax your body and mind. You will want to find a quiet, comfortable spot to practice where you will not be interrupted. You are going to want to totally free your mind. You can do this before sex to cool down your body. This means turn off your phone and computer (or put them on silent), turn off your television, and anything else that is distracting or may cause interruption. You are going to want to quiet your mind first and then move on to relaxing your entire body.

To quiet your mind, you first want to:

■ Lie down in a comfortable spot, use pillows if necessary to make yourself more comfortable.

■ Lie on your back with your arms by your side and close your eyes.

■ You may want to listen to soothing music or relaxation recordings. (Just be sure not to play any music that is distracting or not calming.)

■ Free your mind of any daily concerns; don't worry about that work assignment, feeding the dog or changing the oil in the car. Just let all your worries and concerns slip away for a moment and imagine yourself drifting away.

■ Think of yourself as getting lighter, being held up like a feather in the breeze.

■ Remain this way for as long as you like.

Now, to relax your body, you're going to want to focus on each and every part of your body. This progressive muscle relaxation is similar to getting a full-body massage. You will begin this muscle awareness exercise in your feet and work your way up slowly. Remember, don't rush. Just enjoy the time with yourself.

While lying down on your back, tense up your toes, hold, and then release. Now do your feet; tense your muscles, hold for a moment and then relax. Slowly continue this up your legs. You are now becoming aware of your body and gaining control of your muscles. Work your way up your lower leg and thighs to your butt and genitals. Focus on those muscles and tensing and releasing them.

Breathe naturally as you tense and release the muscles throughout your whole
body, one at a time. Don't forget any part of your sex organs.

Tip 6: Oral Sex

If you want to orally please your woman, you have to understand how first sending the right emotional signals and setting up the right psychological tone can lead to a more fulfilling and rewarding time for her.

Tease her properly

The best way to go down on a woman is not just to open your mouth and jam your tongue right up her pussy. Again, while some chicks dig this, most don't.

You have to send a signal to her that you are going down that way. Maybe you would want to nibble on her tits first, massage the side of her breast, and then lick her tummy.

This buildup psychologically prepares her for the fact that you are going to be putting your head between her legs. The way you do it is also very important. You can't just do this mechanically like you're going through a checklist, or you are painting by numbers. That pretty much strips all the soul out of great oral sex. You have to tease her a bit. Look into her eyes. Have a smile in your eyes and then close your eyes, so there's a bit of mystery. You need to tickle the back of her ears, stimulate the side of her breasts while you're moving your tongue down her body.

Teasing is a very important part of any kind of sex act. It sends a signal to your partner that you're about to do something. It also increases the receptivity of their nerves. You want to reduce your partner into this quivering and highly excited mass of nerves. The more excited she gets, the easier it is for her to cum.

Clitoral stimulation

The secret to clitoral stimulation is that you need to treat her like the way your woman treats your penis when she's blowing it. Seriously. You have to treat it like a small version of your penis. So you need to tease it, suck on it, blow on it, and then you need to move your jaw while you're doing it. Nothing is more boring than just simply licking a clitoris.

Chances are your woman has been around the block a couple of times. She's probably been with at least one other guy, and this is not a completely new experience to her. You have to demonstrate to her that you know how to stimulate a clitoris properly, and this means you need to move your jaw. There has to be some sort of motion there. It's not just your tongue moving. It's also your jaw, which makes your tongue motions stronger and more vigorous. Also, you need to make an "o" with your mouth and suck up the clitoris and then lick it slowly. While you're doing this, you need to be doing things with your hands. You can be looking for that G-spot while you are licking her clitoris, holding her hips down, spreading her legs, massaging her breasts, or even playing with her anus.

Try to stay away from simply licking. You also need to blow, tease - this means touching the tip of her clitoris with the tip of your tongue, and pinching LIGHTLY with your lips.

You have to exercise a lot of variety when you are engaging her clitoris. Otherwise, it's going to be boring, and the sensation would really not be much different from that produced by a vibrator. If a machine can do your job, then your woman doesn't need you.

So do a better job and this means putting her needs ahead of yours in giving oral foreplay the amount of time and energy and passion it deserves.

Finally, make it wet. Use lots of saliva, and don't be afraid of getting messy and slobbering. This will enhance all the sensations, and dryness on her pussy is just unpleasant and sometimes painful. This also gives the appearance of passion, which will turn her on by how into oral sex you are.

Techniques and positions

When it comes to oral stimulation, the best technique would be for her to be comfortable so that she can tune everything else out and just focus on the sensations that you are giving her.

It takes a long time for women to get excited and takes an even longer time for them to cum. You have to position her body so she can reach that point all while remaining comfortable.

The classic position is for her to be on her back with her legs spread. This allows easy access to her breasts, and is comfortable for her.

Another position is for her to sit on your face. You lie on your back and literally pull her on top of you so that her pussy in over your mouth. This can be erotic as she can control the speed and intensity of the oral sex more than she would be able to otherwise.

Finally, I'm a big fan of the woman being on her hands and knees, and you licking her pussy from behind her. This is less comfortable for both of you, but as a short interlude between sex positions, it can be extremely arousing to see her from this position. So how do you know you did the job right? She came.

Tip 7: Try Different Positions

It is very easy for guys to think that all sexual positions are intended and designed primarily for men. live in a male-centered world. As much progress as we have made in terms of gender equality, old mental habits die hard. This is especially true when it comes to sex.

It is easy for guys to pick and choose sexual positions primarily based on how easy it would be for them to get off. This is a bad move if you are trying to take treat of premature ejaculation. Remember, if you want to be a better lover, she has to come first.

You need to make her pleasure a priority if you want to get invited back to the party. If you want her to have a very favorable impression of you, both as a romantic and a sexual partner, you have to make her needs top priority. Instead of automatically picking sexual positions that favor you, focus on what is pleasurable for her.

Finding sex positions to help you and your partner last longer can seem a bit daunting at first. With a bit of foreplay and stimulation, these exciting sex positions can help develop a new approach to intimacy with your partner, while slowing down premature ejaculation. For a longer, lasting experience in the bedroom that the both of you will enjoy, here are the best sex positions to help slow things down and maximize pleasure for her. The good news is that, the internet being the internet, there are tons of research materials you can check out, when looking into these positions. Many of these research resources have photos, so you don't have to scratch your head as to what these positions look like. There are more than enough resources out there to help you pull off these sexual positions like a pro.

Cowgirl

This position has been said to be one of the best sexual positions if you want to know how to treat premature ejaculation.

Cowgirl position is pretty straightforward. The woman straddles the man while he is flat on his back. The great thing about the cowgirl position is that it maximizes control for the woman.

To orgasm, women have a certain pattern and rhythm. They need to build up slowly, and then pick up pace and scale. Guys sometimes completely lose sight of this fact and, eventually either pump too hard, pump too slow, or do something that prevents the woman from climaxing. You can get her close to it, but it only takes a few missteps and the opportunity closes.

Now, why is this the best position to help you last longer in bed? With this position, you are able to relax. One of the key answers about how to treat premature ejaculation is about relaxing your body and mind. This "cowgirl" position takes away the stress for you to perform. Instead, what you do is merely to lie down and let her take charge. When your body is relaxed, you will be in greater control of your arousal and that will slow down your ejaculation.

Reversed Cowgirl

This is another sexual position that holds the answer to how to treat premature ejaculation.

In this position, your female partner stays on top of you but with her back facing you. You may easily stretch your hand to caress her breasts and enjoy the fund and pleasure of the act. Like the first position, this position allows you to relax your body and prevent premature ejaculation without any extra effort.

Spooning

Slow and steady wins the race and this position is sure to make you and your partner both feel like winners. If you think that it is romantic to lie down at the back of your partner and cuddle, you will find spooning sex very sexy. This is because it has the emotional intimacy of spooning while you are penetrating her. Have your partner lay on her side, as you lay down behind her facing the same direction as you enter her. Not only does this position allow you to take things slower, it gives you access to touch and caress your partner while maintaining a rhythm that is sure to please both of you.

The same applies to your partner. Your partner feels appreciated, loved, caressed, and sexually gratified. Again, this is primarily psychological because, in terms of clitoral contact, spooning is kind of a difficult position, to maximize clitoral or G-spot contact. It does happen, though.

Sideways cowgirl

This is for the more athletic women out there. Cowgirl and reverse cowgirl positions are pretty straightforward because you are basically just sitting on your partner's penis. However, sideways cowgirl involves the woman sitting at a 90 degree angle to her partner. Instead of straddling him straight on, she sits to the side.

The great about the sideways cowgirl is that it increases clitoral stimulation and maximizes control, because the woman is still on top. It does take a lot more effort to perfect. But, if you are looking for your female partner to come regularly and predictably, this is the position you should encourage her to take. It takes an adventurous woman to try this because it does take quite a bit of effort.

Side By Side

This position is where you and your female partner lie down "side by side" with her back facing you. Her hips should be pressed against your groin while you enter her from behind.

How to treat premature ejaculation with this position? Well, like the above positions, this position gives you a lot of control over your stimulation and arousal level which helps you to prevent premature ejaculation.

By lying down, you take away the stress and tension exerted on your arms and legs. You are also able to control the thrusting speed, depth and intensity.

This is also a great position as you can slow down your thrusting anytime and lean over to kiss her or caress her breasts. This will help diverting your attention from your own pleasure and keep any untimely ejaculation at bay.

Face to Face

When your lover sits on your lap, she assumes control of the intensity and speed of your love-making.

This position still allows you to be intimate, and you may distract yourself with kissing and caressing during intercourse. The back and forth motion may be easier for you to tolerate for longer than up and down movements, so experiment and see how you can up the ante over a gradual period rather than rushing towards climax.

Chair seat

Find a sturdy chair or sofa that will allow you and your partner to be comfortable. Have your partner face away from you as she lowers herself onto your lap. Use your arms to help navigate her down as she slowly moves up and down. Have fun varying the speed between you and your partner for an irresistible sensation that is sure to slow you down but speed her up.

Standing

It is all about positioning. The great thing about sex while standing is that there is a lot of emotional urgency to it.

Usually, people who have sex standing are those people who don't have much time to get off. There is this sense of danger. There is this sense of surprise. There is that improvised atmosphere to the air when you are doing it while standing up. While, physically speaking, this does not necessarily get her off, it does, psychologically, get her excited. Since sex is 90% psychological and 10% physical, this position definitely deserves to be at the top of the list.

Doggie style

Doggie style is pretty straightforward. It is one of the most basic sexual positions. It is also one of the most effective and popular. The reason why it is very popular is because it pleasures both men and women.

It allows for maximum clitoral stimulation, especially if you reach over her hips and rub her clit from behind. It also maximizes vaginal penetration. Whether you are trying to get your partner to orgasm through stimulating her clitoris, or you want to get her off by exciting her G-spot, doggie style is it. Also, doggie style isn't very complicated. You don't have to be a rocket scientist to pull this off.

The more positions you experiment, the higher chances for you to find the best sexual position that gives you greater control over your arousal and ejaculation. In addition to that, trying various styles and positions will add more spice and fun to your entire sexual experience.

Tip 8: PC Muscle Exercise

Muscle exercises that deal with issues related to the sexual organ are most commonly attributed to women than to men. These muscle exercises are known as **Kegel exercises** and are mostly recommended to women who have just given birth. It involves consciously contracting the muscle that is known as the pubococcygeus (PC) muscle. This is also the same muscle that women employ to hold their pee in.

Apparently, the same muscle is also present in the male reproductive tract and performs the same function. Experts believe that men with lifelong premature ejaculation would benefit a lot by simply performing the Kegel exercises daily for up to 12 weeks. *This has been proven effective in a study done by a team of researchers under the direction of Dr Antonio Pastore of the Sapienza University of Rome.* Further study still needs to be done on the matter. However, the results were conclusive enough to be presented at a convention of Urologists in Stockholm, Sweden.

Men who are experiencing premature ejaculation can follow the steps that Dr Pastore's subjects were advised to do.

■ The first step is to try to identify the PC muscle. In anatomical illustrations, this muscle lies horizontally extending from the pubic bone to the tail bone (coccyx). When a man is standing upright, the PC muscle is shaped slightly like a hammock. You can identify it within yourself by sitting in a relaxed position.

■ You then need to try to contract the muscles around the back of the pelvic area in the same manner as when you try to contract it in trying to hold a fart or fecal matter in. The muscle that moves during this process is the same PC muscle that you need to exercise in order to address premature ejaculation. you need to contract this muscle tightly for a few seconds and then slowly loosen it up again. You should then let the muscle rest for about 4-5 seconds and then repeat the contractions. You can start with one or two contractions for the first couple of days until you build up to 10 daily contractions.

■ Once you have grown accustomed to slowly contracting the PC muscle for several repetitions, the next goal is to hold each of the contractions tightly for up to 10 seconds. Aside from sitting down, men can also perform the Kegel exercises while standing. Another option is to lie down flat on your backs with your knees placed slightly apart. *According to the study, reliable results will only start to show after doing the daily Kegel exercise for 3 months.*

According to Dr Pastore's peers, doing the Kegel exercises is advantageous not just because it helps men gain better muscular control. It also has a huge impact on men's psychological well-being. That ' s because men who are suffering from premature ejaculation are the same ones who handle their own therapy. Experts believe that the process helps enhance their self-esteem and provides them with a welcome diversion against stressful thoughts.

Another variation of the Kegel exercise is the Reverse Kegel. This is a relatively new concept and not a lot of experts recommend it yet. It basically involves doing the exact opposite of the Kegel exercises. So instead of contracting the muscles, they are stimulated into a relaxed state. Familiarity with the standard Kegel exercises is necessary in order for men to be able to successfully pull off the reverse.

Otherwise, you may have a hard time identifying not just the PC muscle but also the bulbocavernosus (BC) muscle. Once you have familiarized the normal Kegel exercises, you can then proceed with the following steps for the Reverse Kegel:

■ Sit in a relaxed position.

■ Gently try to relax the muscles around the anal area in a simulation of the same movements when trying to push fecal matter or pee out. Note: be sure to do it gently if you don't want an 'accident' to come rushing out. Do the first two steps for several repetitions. One way to confirm if you're doing it correctly is if the lower abdominal muscles get tense during the simulation. Try to do the reverse Kegel exercises again and be sure to observe what happens in the lower abdominal area. If it is tensed while the coccygeal muscles are relaxing, then it is time for the next step:

■ Combine the reverse Kegel exercise with breathing exercises that draw breath directly to and from the diaphragm instead of the chest. This should be easy to accomplish if the first two steps were done correctly. Just breathe in deeply until the belly gets distended. Then slowly breathe the air out while simulating the act of peeing or pushing poop out. Doing this step can help men in identifying the specific muscles that they need to control.

■ Once they master the third step, the next thing to do is to try to simulate a relaxed state in the coccygeal muscles without relying on the assistance of the abdominal muscles. This means trying to do the reverse Kegel without doing the diaphragm breathing exercises.

The fourth step may be a little more difficult to accomplish and not everyone can be successful at it. One expert recommendation is to visualize the muscles around the coccygeal area. Try to imagine each muscle slowly opening up as you slowly try to relax it.

Kegel and reverse Kegel exercises each have their own functions during sex. The normal Kegel exercises should only be performed once you reach a point wherein you can no longer control the ejaculation at all. Otherwise, you might end up pushing the PC muscles too hard and end up ejaculating prematurely instead of achieving the opposite. I recommend doing normal Kegels at the beginning of intercourse because it can help enhance an erection.

On the other hand, reverse Kegels should be performed while in the middle of foreplay. This is believed to help men with premature ejaculation last longer during sex. That ' s because the contraction of the PC muscle tightens a man ' s arousal becomes more pronounced. This is why doing normal Kegels during foreplay can aggravate premature ejaculation instead of alleviating it. But when you have mastered the art of relaxing the PC and BC muscles through the reverse Kegel, you can consciously control it during sex so that it wouldn't contract tightly early on.

Tip 9: Pleasuring Your Partner Without Penetration

Men who ejaculate almost as soon as penetration occurs should at least learn how to use foreplay to pleasure their partners effectively, even without penetration. You can make use of these moves in pleasuring your partner while you are still waiting on the techniques above to take effect. These moves ensure that your partner are going to have as many orgasms as possible without penetration. The foreplay moves include:

Squeeze, knead, and tease all of her G-spots. Contrary to the prevailing belief, the clitoris is not the only G-spot in women ' s bodies. There are 4 other spots that you should focus your attention on during foreplay. These are the:

1. Neck
2. Arm
3. Thigh

4. Foot

■ **Use sex toys.** People ' s interest in sex toys reached a peak when E.L. James ' book Fifty Shades of Grey first came out. All this interest is justified by the fact that sex toys are highly effective in spicing up your time in the bedroom. Toys such as vibrators and dildos can help women achieve orgasm without actual penile penetration. What ' s more, men can expect to give their partners multiple orgasms if they learn to use the toys correctly.

■ **Talk dirty.** Women who read a lot of romance novels may have gotten one wrong impression: men grunt, moan, or be vocal about their pleasures during sex. However, this is far from the truth since about 90% of menare quiet during intercourse. If you're among the 90%, then it's time to up the ante a little bit. Grunting or moaning may feel uncomfortable especially during foreplay, but you should still do it nonetheless. The next best option for being vocally active is to do some dirty talking. You can talk dirty in and out of the bedroom, especially if the couple have already established a trusting relationship.

■ **Touch your partner body.** Some men may have learned their foreplay moves from watching porn videos. This is unfortunate since porn rarely focuses on the woman's actual pleasure, which means the women in the videos don't get touched much. A woman's body has more sensitive zones than a man's does. This is proven by the fact that women have several pleasure spots (G-spots). Touch these spots with gentle teasing caresses and then follow it up with your mouth.

These pleasure-driven tips not only help you delay their ejaculation by a few more precious minutes. Mastering these moves also ensures that you can get rid of your performance anxiety so you can relax and fully enjoy the experience.

Tip 10: Cool Draw Method

Cool draw method also called as Testicle Breathing. Massage your testicles until you get slight feeling of sexual energy. Now take a deep breath and simultaneously pull upwards using the muscles around the testicles and anus.

As you do so, use your mind to visualize the sexual energy from your testicles being drawn out towards your anus. Then exhale slowly and relax. Repeat this breathing exercise a few times. While breathing, you should focus on the transfer of your sexual energy from your testicles across you perineum and towards the anus. You should eventually feel a tingling sensation moving across this path. press your tongue Once this happens, continue to breathe slowly and focus on that energy. Move it away from your perineum via the anus all the way up your spine. You should be able to feel that tingling sensation moving through your body towards your head.

It might take up to 10 minutes. But, eventually the tingling will reach your head. At this point, you can press your tongue to the roof your mouth and feel the energy slipping away down the front of your body. The whole technique is based around visualization and the use of the mind, as premature ejaculation is often a mental problem.

You can practice this technique several times until you begin to master it. Then, during sexual sessions, make use of it. This will help to draw the sexual energy away from your penis and testicles, freeing the pressure in these areas. Thus, allowing you to have sex for longer periods of time.

Tip 11: Big Draw Method

In big draw method you move energy from the genital region along the spine and circulate it around the body.

How to do it? While you are near to orgasm simply squeeze your PC muscles. Now blood go away from genitals. This method decreases your arousal and the same time you draw the energy from the genital area by imagining an energy traveling up your spine into your brain.

By using big draw method you can achieve full body orgasm.

Tip 12: Thrusting Technique

In many cases, when a man and woman have sex, the accepted way of intercourse is by simply thrusting in and out, no matter what sex position is utilized. Through this motion, the man is generally able to achieve an orgasm and ejaculate, while the woman more often than not, feels discomfort or pain and without any orgasm at all, thus leaving both parties feeling frustrated and disappointed at the end of every session.

The reason why this occurs is because of the monotonous, ineffective in-and-out thrusting. In addition, many men have been led to believe that the deeper they go and the faster they thrust, the better off their partner is. The truth is that by simply thrusting in and out, you will find that your penis is by-passing some of the most sensitive areas of your partner's vagina, and in many cases, you are doing nothing more than causing discomfort and pain to your woman every time the tip of your penis hits against her cervix wall without any type of control.

In this section, I will be sharing with you one extremely powerful thrusting technique you can try with your partner tonight. This technique is not only effective at increasing your performance and making you last longer, but it also has other stunning benefits that can help both a man and woman to achieve a very fulfilling lovemaking session.

The Next Time you Make Love to Her, Try the Following Technique:

■ Once both of you are turned on, and your partner is sufficiently lubricated, and you are about to penetrate her, do not insert your penis all the way inside.

■ Instead, insert just a little more than the head of your penis only. When you begin to thrust, keep your strokes very shallow. In other words, your penis should not move more than an inch in either direction when you are thrusting. In addition, you should keep these movements slow and deliberate. The idea is to ensure that your penis is at all times remaining near the entrance of your partner's vaginal canal while you are thrusting.

This will be extremely arousing for your partner. That is because the area around the entrance of the vaginal canal is the most pleasurably sensitive for your partner. Think about it, both the clitoris and g-spot are situated near and at the entrance of a woman's vaginal canal.

You Can Also Add Some Variations to your Strokes

For example, after a few short strokes, you can then go ahead and give one deep thrust, or two, or three, depending on the mood. You can also add variation in terms of how you angle your member.

Now and then, you could stimulate your partner's g-spot by pushing the tip of your penis against the upper wall of your partner's vaginal canal.

Here are Some Extra Benefits you can Both Gain from this Thrusting Technique:

1.   It allows the both of you more time to truly enjoy the intercourse session as you are forced to slow down and appreciate the sensations you are feeling.

2.   This is a great way to last longer. Because you are forced to slow down and not thrust too deeply or too vigorously, it becomes easier for you to learn and understand your sensations and climax thresholds in terms of when you feel you might need to ejaculate. This is because you are minimizing the amount of muscles that are being used in your body during thrusting, thus avoiding higher sensations of arousal that can occur through vigorous and deep thrusting.

3.   If you have a larger than average penis, you can also benefit from this technique. That is because you are forced to slow down when thrusting, thus having more control when going for deeper thrusts, which in turn prevents you

from accidentally hitting too hard against your partner's cervix wall. If on the other hand you feel you have a smaller than average penis, this is an excellent technique that allows you to focus less on worrying about size and more on actually stimulating the areas that matters most for many women.

4.   For your partner, this technique is a great way to initiate intercourse because it helps her to relax and to become aroused so that she can gradually become ready for deep thrusting.

Keep in Mind that Not All Sex Positions are Perfect for this Type of Thrusting Technique

One of the best positions to accomplish this technique effectively is by having your partner lie on her back at the edge of the bed while you stand or kneel on the floor at the side of the bed. The idea is to find a position that allows you to move slowly, shallowly, and to be able to do all of this without losing balance or feeling like you are flexing every muscle in your body. This is especially important if you are suffering from premature ejaculation. You need to make sure that the posture of your body is in a completely relaxed state.

It also depends on what you want to do during the time you are thrusting. For example, if you are looking for space between yourself and your partner so that you can freely use your hands to stimulate other areas of her body, then you would want a sex position that does not have you lying right on top of your partner, such as the missionary position. Instead, you could modify the missionary position so that you are sitting upright and kneeling on the bed. To make things more comfortable for your partner, you could place a pillow underneath her butt.

By introducing effective techniques like the one mentioned in this chapter when having intercourse, you will be ensuring that both your partner and yourself will be experiencing a more satisfying lovemaking session every time.

Chapter 6: 10 Habits That Can Boost Your Sex Life

1. Eat Healthy.

Sex drives of any individual varies considerably and people who are worried about a low sex drive can help to increase libido through eating a healthy and well balanced diet which includes all the minerals and vitamins and nutrients required to keep your body in tiptop condition. Here we look at some of the elements of food which help to promote a healthy sex life and those foods which can have an adverse affect on your overall libido.

There are some nutrients in our diets which are critically important to our overall sexual health. A good example is zinc in our diets being required to promote healthy and productive sperm. It is additionally particularly important in the development of our reproductive organs. Zinc deficiencies in our bodies can lead to infertility and in some cases premature ejaculation. The highest zinc containing foods are oysters and it is therefore no surprise that their legendary status as a sexual aphrodisiac has some degree of truth to it. Pumpkin seeds, crab and offal products are also excellent sources of the zinc vitamin.

Avoid smoking and drinking

It has long been known that smoking and alcohol consumption have been known to suppress the sex drives of individuals who smoke and drink to excess. Smoking increases the risk of suffering from hardening of the arteries and a narrowing of the penile artery is the common root cause of impotence in older men. The risk of suffering from impotence can be reduced by ceasing smoking and eating plenty of antioxidants in your daily diet. In terms of alcohol, constituents within the hops used in the beer making process also are utilised in medicines to reduce the sex drive of men. These constituent hops are therefore consumed ordinarily when drinking beer which has been proven to reduce the sex drive.

High caffeine intakes ordinarily found in tea, coffee and chocolate have also been known to reduce sex drive. High blood pressure, high cholesterol and various prescription drugs have also been seen to be playing a part in the lowering of individual sex drives.

Despite the abundance of products claiming to have significant aphrodisiac effects, there is currently no scientific evidence to substantiate the majority of these supplements. Common examples include powdered rhino horn, Spanish fly to name but a few. There is a degree of scientific evidence to suggest that ginseng may help to increase low sex drives.

It is widely believed that including eggs, wheat germ and broccoli which are all high in vitamins E, will help to maintain a healthy sex drive although it is noted there is currently no scientific evidence to support this.

Therefore, if you are looking to increase your sex drive, include zinc rich foods in your diet and avoid excessive amounts of caffeine and nicotine and try to keep your alcohol consumption to a low-level. **You can refer to chapter 4 for more detail on healthy food to boost your sex life.**

2. Appreciate That Not Every Intimate Contact Has to Lead to Full Intercourse

I often hear people say that they avoid being physically affectionate when they are too tired for sex because they don't want to risk disappointing their partner who takes any sign of closeness as sexual encouragement.

As time passes a couple often discover that they have different sex drives. One person may have a higher sex drive than the other, but it is possible to find positive ways to accommodate both people in a healthy sexual relationship.

Discuss how you feel about sex and intimacy when you are both calm and relaxed. Explain that the times when you don't want full sex do not mean rejection or lack of sexual interest in your partner. Be clear that you want to cuddle, pet and be playful, but not always take it all the way.

3. Talking Openly With Your Partner

As I've said before, Premature ejaculation isn't just about you. It also affects your partner, not just in how you're able to satisfy her sexually, but also in how she responds to, and deals with, your Premature ejaculation. Simply put, Premature ejaculation is a relationship issue.

If you've already had a frank discussion with your partner about Premature ejaculation, congratulations. You're already way ahead of most guys, who would probably rather deconstruct the latest episode of Gossip Girl than talk about Premature ejaculation. Sure, you might feel uncomfortable or embarrassed to bring it up, but this is one of the most important conversations you and your partner will ever have.

In fact, if you don't talk about Premature ejaculation with your partner, you can make it worse. She may not understand what's happening and why and will feel confused. if your partner doesn't already know you suffer from premature ejaculation then it's time she did because;

■　She either already thinks you're just a loser in bed OR

■　She thinks that she isn't doing it for you and you're just want to get sex over with as quickly as possible

■　Neither of these two scenarios are true, so why should you let your relationship go on like that? It's time to tell her the truth!

Why Should She Need to Know How to Delay Ejaculation?

That's a fair question. We're men, and our ego's and strength of character may make us think we can deal with the problem ourselves, but like many other things in life, that just isn't true. You need your partner on your side through this problem, and if she is totally clueless as to what is going on, then things will just get worse as time goes on.

This will mean arguments, fights, and at the very worst end, separation and divorce. All because you are too proud to tell her you suffer from premature ejaculation? Break the silence now, before it's too late.

I Know I Need to Share, But I'm Embarrassed to Tell Her

It can't be any more embarrassing than the situation that you're in just now. Your woman thinking that you're just a "one minute wonder" in the bedroom, and can't satisfy her even if you tried. She's your partner, your lover, and if you're lucky, she's also your soul mate, so give her the respect that she deserves and just tell her what is going on.

Where is the Best Place to Break This To Her?

Don't think of it that way, this is a situation that is not directly your fault, so dump those negative feelings about your premature ejaculation problem right now, they will do you no good whatsoever.

The best place to tell her would be in the place you feel most comfortable, perhaps in the house, or maybe take her for a short walk and tell her about the problem.

- How long you've had the problem
- What you think has caused the problem
- That you're not going to let it beat you

Of course, when it comes to communicating about sex, there's often a gap between what we want to say and how we end up saying it, and even the gentlest of words can come off as confrontational. Criticism, expressed or perceived harshly, is the sexual kiss of death. So if you can, try to express your desires as a positive turn-on rather than a negative turn-off. Here is a few tips

- **Get closer.** For guys with Premature ejaculation, that means using intimate moments outside the bedroom to start a conversation. For example, as you come out of a kiss with your partner, say something like, "*I love kissing you and being with you, and really want you to enjoy it when we're* *together. I know sometimes sex can feel rushed, but I really want to make an effort to slow things down and appreciate every second with you."* You can use these little bursts of conversation following an intimate moment to reveal your Premature ejaculation and your feelings about it.

■ **Talk "by" her not "to" her.** If you're too uncomfortable talking about sex face to face, you've got other options. Anthropologists have long observed that women are "face-to-face" communicators, while men do so "side by side." This means that women are much more comfortable with direct eye contact, which probably has a lot to do with the female history of nursing, cuddling, and generally fawning over their infants all the while staring lovingly into those big baby eyes. Some men, on the other hand, find direct eye contact extremely confrontational. It may be easier for you to have your talk while you're taking a walk, driving, shopping, or watching TV together.

■ **Make it fun.** Extended foreplay is also the ideal time to have an intimate conversation. Try to get in the habit of sharing your fantasies and desires with each other, talking about what works and what doesn't work. By extending foreplay, you create the perfect "time-zone" for talking about sex because as arousal heightens, our inhibitions lower due to a potent neurochemical cocktail unique to sexual arousal. It becomes easier to give feedback about how good something feels, or conversely if something could feel better. It's also easier to share a naughty thought or fantasy. The point is that talking about sex should be sexy and having a con-structive conversation can actually be part of foreplay. Guys with Premature ejaculation can take advantage of this process: For example, tell your partner that you have a fantasy or sexy dream that features the sex script that works best for you—in most cases, that's oral sex. Or, suggest mutual masturbation and taking turns as giver or receiver to prolong pleasure for both of you.

Clear the Air, And Strengthen Your Bond!

Once you have spoken with her and let her know exactly what is going on, then she will respect you and love you more than ever for both your honesty and trust in her. And believe me, these are both good things when it comes to forming a long lasting and strong bond with each other.

The chances are, she will already be aware that there is a problem in your relationship, so this will be a relief to hear that she isn't at fault or doesn't turn you on anymore.

4. Understand that Woman Have Private Sex Drive

Unfortunately, most guys know more about what's under the hood of a car than the hood of a clitoris. We're woefully uninformed about female sexuality—not just the physical aspects, but the emotional aspects as well. I'm not going to spend too much time on the intricacies of satisfying a woman, but making sure your partner is satisfied is clearly crucial for guys with - Be premature ejaculation. Here are the basics you should know.

Emotion

Generally, before a woman can get aroused, she has to experience desire. In this way, female sexuality is different than male sexuality. For most men, all it takes is a little visual stimulation to get us in the mood for sex. That's why men are the predominant consumers of porn and why something like Viagra works so well for men, but not for women.

Men are more easily aroused, and arousal is more directly linked to desire. Female sexuality is a little more complex. In fact, one of the main differences between male and female sexuality is that guys don't need to feel emotionally connected to the person we're having sex with in order to want to have sex. There's actually scientific research to support the observation that women tend to feel sexual desire towards those men for whom they feel an emotional connection. It could be a function of evolution. Men have a virtually unlimited supply of sperm to propagate, but women have precious few eggs to be fertilized. So they're going to be choosier about whom they have sex with, and part of that choosiness is the need to feel emotionally connected.

These days, of course, not every woman wants you to fertilize her eggs and many couples use some sort of birth control. But for many women, the need for an emotional connection hasn't ebbed. This means the first thing you can do to get a woman in the mood for sex is to make a strong emotional connection outside the bedroom. Men with premature ejaculation tend to focus on the fact that they can't last long, so they idealize a vision of sex in which they can last longer and often emphasize aspects that are less important. Most guys with premature ejaculation don't think as much about the emotional connection, because they're so concerned with performance issues. If you want to share a healthy, satisfying sex life with your partner, that needs to change.

What's a simple way to make an emotional connection? Try hugging for 20 seconds. It sounds simple and 20 seconds can be a long time to hug but studies have shown that's about the amount of time it takes for women to produce significant levels of oxytocin, also known as the cuddle hormone. Oxytocin is stimulated via touch, and is directly correlated with a sense of connection and well-being. Women produce way more oxytocin than men, and while that's not to say that you won't enjoy the hug, too (as well as other forms of touch that stimulate oxytocin), it may not deliver the same sense of emotional connection. As we mentioned earlier in this section, many women need to experience an emotional connection in order to experience desire, and the oxytocin connection may well be the reason why.

Anxiety

As you just learned, a woman's biggest sex organ is her brain. But remember, to turn her on, you need to help her turn her brain off. Brain responsible for processing fear, anxiety, and emotion slowed down significantly in women but not men as they became aroused. That's powerful evidence that women need to let go of fear and anxiety to climax.

As I've said before, women don't have the female equivalent of a point of ejaculatory inevitability, and they can lose an orgasm even as it's happening. **Let me repeat:** If you want your partner to get turned on, you have to help her turn off her brain. That means leaving your worries outside the bedroom, which can be challenging but not impossible for couples dealing with premature ejaculation.

Fantasy

Research shows that people with active fantasy lives are more sexually satisfied, more sexually responsive and more adventurous regarding sex in general. There's a difference between sharing a fantasy and actually acting one out, and sharing a naughty thought or two might be all you need to get the ball rolling. Studies have found that women tend to fantasize more than men during sex, which helps them escape reality and facilitate that important process of "turning off" the brain that we discussed in last point.

Fantasy is a cousin of dreaming and as neuroscientist Mark Solms, a leading expert in the field of sleep research, explains, *"Dreaming does for the brain what Saturday morning cartoons do for the kids: It keeps them suf-ficiently entertained so that the serious players in the household can get needed recovery time. Without such diversion, the brain would be urging us up and out into the world to keep it fully engaged."* Guys with premature ejaculation can rely on fantasy as a powerful tool to get a woman closer to orgasm without having to rely on physical stimulation.

Anatomy

The brain may be a woman's biggest sex organ, but it isn't the only one. To satisfy your partner, you have to know your way around the geography of her vulva, too. That includes the northern tippy-top of the clitoral glans (the "love-button," so to speak), to the western and eastern boundaries of the labia minora (her inner lips) to the southernmost regions of the perineum (the smooth expanse of skin just below the vaginal entrance) and anus. Understanding a woman's body is crucial to helping her achieve orgasm: With more than 18 parts, twice as many nerve endings as the penis, and the enviable ability to produce multiple orgasms, the clitoris is the in-disputable powerhouse of female sexuality. The vast majority of nerve endings that contribute to female orgasm are located on surface of the vulva and do not require vaginal penetration. That's why applying pressure and rhythm to the vulva, and specifically the clitoris, is more important than constantly thrusting or switching positions. In fact, many intercourse positions don't stimulate her clitoris at all—and won't give her an orgasm. So get cliterate!

Remember, premature ejaculation is less of a problem if you can satisfy a woman, regardless of how that happens. Many men with premature ejaculation become skilled at oral sex. As I have described in Chapter 5, oral sex isn't just the most consistent way to give a woman an orgasm, it takes the pressure off your penis and allows you to slow down and observe.

It's imperative that you focus more on satisfying your partner, period, and less on whether her orgasm occurs through intercourse. Partners of men with premature ejaculation are more likely to cheat, especially if they are not

achieving orgasms in other ways. Many women will say that it's okay, and generally women seem more accepting of sexual experiences that don't always include orgasms, but this is really the exception rather than rule, and we should not get into the mindset of diminishing the importance of the female orgasm as part of the overall experience of sex. Your partner is less likely to be angry and aggravated about your premature ejaculation if she's feeling fulfilled. She still might be frustrated that sex needs to happen in a certain way or that she's limited in pleasuring you, but in general she'll be more supportive. Give your partner an orgasm and you shift premature ejaculation from Code Red to a more tolerable situation for you both.

5. Always Touch Her Feelings Before You Touch Her Body

As women take a longer time to get aroused than men and this reality is what makes men absolutely impractical about how to make women totally satisfied and fulfilled during sex. It is imperative that you spend sufficient time on foreplay and make a women heat up and excited to an intense pitch before you even begin to focus about on your own pleasure and satisfaction. If you do not have patience and do not take it slow and easy, your woman will have no interest in you and much anticipated explosive sex will fly out of the window.

Tease her, entice her and build up her inner passions in order to achieve better results. Give her enough gratification so that she will think you to be a sex god, and she will feel fortunate to be your girlfriend. If you wish to pick up some tips on how to make a woman go crazy for you, here are some tactics that you can use tonight...

Almost Touching

While you're speaking to her, softly place your hands on her shoulders and arms, and then move smoothly down. The strategy is not to caress her, but to let your hands remain, or flit around, her skin. This will augment and enhance the sexual tensions as her need for your touch will increase. You may be astounded as she could be initiating love making after you get her aroused sufficiently.

Taking In the Scent of Her

By targeting sexually sensitive sections on her body and then, believe it or not, sniffing them, you can drive a woman totally crazy.

Breathe in the scent of her hair and simultaneously breathe warm air down her neck and back. Then, lightly blow upon her nipples, and keep teasing her by going to lick them but stopping short. Believe me, you'll have her completely turned on and ready for anything in no time.

Talk and Tease

As women are natural inspired thinkers, you can utilize this quality to your advantage by exciting and teasing her imagination all through foreplay (or prior to that). Just talk to her in a teasing way to make her feel deeply aware of your being there with her. Be craft and clever and entice her to want to get closer to you simply by describing in detail what you desire to do to her. With some measure of luck, it will be her initiating wild sex with you after a dinner date or a night out at the movies.

Tease Her Relentlessly. Move as close as you can to her without actually touching her body. If you stop just before making contact, it really builds up the anticipation.

One way to put this method to good is use to move the tip of your tongue to within millimeters of her clitoris. She'll be expecting to feel the satisfaction of your warm tongue, and when you don't give it to her she may just turn the tables and become the aggressive one in bed.

Breathing Therapy

Press together your lips and let out a steady stream of breath aimed at at her exposed skin. This stream of air will be indicative of your 'touch' and you can do this action just about anywhere; while seated next to her on the couch while enjoying your favorite T.V. show, as you're watching a movie, or even as you're walking together.

6. Build a Safer Sex Arsenal

Sex is the most pleasing activity of our life. Its attractions and rewards are enormous. It is not untrue to say 'no sex no life.' Life without sex will certainly become a dull and bore routine, meaningless and fruitless. While this natural process is full of such tremendous excitements, it is also full of life threatening hazards.

We all know the alarming situation of sexually transmitted diseases, where AIDS or HIV is more dominant and deadly. The toll is rising fast since people seek illegitimate sexual outlets where you do not know your sexual partners' standing (perhaps you are not the only one having sex with him or her); you do not know with what diseases he or she is suffering from. The answer to such a question is, avoid unprotected sex with new partners or while having sex outside the marriage boundary. But how safe is the use of condom, is it 100% safe?

The safest mean, of course, is the sexual relations between a husband and wife. This is what we consider the natural limits. When we cross any limit set by the nature, it will certainly punish us. Anal sex and sex between two identical sexes, all are like crossing the nature's boundary that invites certain punishments. As a result of crossing the limits set up by the nature, we find the rising cases of sexually transmitted diseases, and the life threatening hazards of AIDS or HIV.

Unprotected sex invites negative consequences, such as incurable diseases (HIV, AIDS, Hepatitis, and Herpes), curable diseases (Syphilis, Chlamydia, Gonnorhea), Infertility, Cervical cancer, unwanted pregnancy and other complications associated with its termination, etc.

It is not fair and logical to advice to stay away from sex to save oneself from getting any sexually transmitted disease. Sex is a great gift of the nature which has to be enjoyed as much as possible. You can't stay away from sex and yet find the life enjoyable. Of course legitimate sex between a wife and husband is the safest mean to enjoy with this precious gift, but it is, of course, not always possible. We should, therefore, try to find more tips and methods for safer sex.

Adopting preventive measures like condoms

The use of condom prevents you from acquiring many sexually transmitted diseases; but this method is not 100% safe, be careful. Put on the condom carefully; pinch the air out of the top when putting it on otherwise the condom can break. If you have to use lubricants, use a water-based one, otherwise other lubricating media like body lotion, butter, petroleum jelly, etc can break down latex condoms.

Use condoms of very high quality and only certified ones. Ensure condom's health (validity, proper storage, etc).

If your lover gives you a hard time about wearing a condom, here are some good responses and excellent reasons why you need to use one.

Him: I don't think condoms are romantic.

Her: Just let me show you how romantic condoms can be.

Him: You don't trust me, do you?

Her: It's not a matter of trust; it's a matter of health.

Him: I don't like to use condoms.

Her: I don't have sex without them.

Him: I haven't had sex with anyone in years so I know I'm clean.

Her: Thanks for being so honest, but let's use one anyway.

Him: I can't feel anything when I wear a condom.

Her: Let me provide you with some extra stimulation.

Him: I know I'll lose my erection by the time I get it on.

Her: Here, let me put it on for you with my mouth.

Him: I'm only going to use a condom this once.

Her: Once is all it takes.

Him: Sorry, I don't have one.

Her: That's ok. I do.

Him: How come you have condoms on you? Did you plan to have sex with me?

Her: I made sure I had some because I really care about you.

Him: Forget it. I'm not going to use a condom.

Her: Fine. Then let's not have sex until we can work out our differences.

Cutting down on the number of partners

Even though monogamy does not provide a 100 % guarantee from infections, you can at least mitigate the possibilities of contracting them from an infected partner. Hence, try to limit the number of partners you have a sexual relationship with.

Undergoing regular medical screening

Even if you have not indulged in sex recently, it is a good idea to undergo a medical screening to make sure there are no signs like tumors or warts, indicative of infections and diseases.

Taking a promise to not to play with either your health or your partner's

You have to respect your partner's feelings and emotions and can never play with their health. Hence, discussing openly with your partner about the intended goals of the sexual relationship goes a long way in maintaining a good understanding between both of you, which in turn helps in adopting a safe sexual relationship, free from fear or risk. A diligent and conscientious attitude towards the maintenance of good overall sexual health is also necessary in this aspect.

Refraining from going overboard

Too much of anything is always risky and unpleasant; so is it with sex too. Make sure you stick to your predetermined plan when indulging in sex. Never commit the mistake of combining practices like smoking or drinking with sex- the results may just be the opposite of what you desired to get from sex.

Other tips

■ Avoid having sex with completely strange people. Remember, condoms are not 100% safe.

■ While engaging in oral sex, do not forget the hygienic side. Both he and she must clean the private parts before the act.

■ Avoid anal sex at all (don't forget nature's punishment).

■ Avoid using uncertified oils (in case of vaginal dryness), and other substances for lubrication; this is essential to prevent fungal and other infections.

■ Avoid having sex with sex workers, for the very apparent reasons which we all know. Do not rely on condoms.

Sex is a natural drive which, if done properly while taking care of the necessary precautions, can give you the pleasure which no other act can offer.

7. Do Kegel Exercises Daily

Do you remember the time when you had to pee like a racehorse, but you had to hold it in? Do you remember the time when you were driving and you felt the need to urinate, but you can't find a gas station with a bathroom so you had to hold it in? Well, the skills you learned holding it in can really pay off.

When you are preventing yourself from peeing, you are exercising muscles in your groin area, that can come in handy when it comes to sex. Just as you can hold in urine with these exercises, you can prevent premature ejaculation. That is right. You can hold in your orgasm long enough for your partner to come. When you flex that muscle for a few sets of 20 a day, you will be able to control your orgasm essentially. When you feel the orgasm bubbling up, you will simply be able to flex your kegels, and keep it at bay.

This is why male porn stars hang on to their job for such a long time. They can manage their ejaculation. Men have a better ability of doing this than women.

When you have such strong kegels, it also gives you harder, and higher quality erections because you literally have the ability to pump blood into your penis at will.

8. Avoid Porn

Porn is a massive issue for men today. There is so much about. It's so easy to

access. Porn's advocates would have us believe that porn is sex positive,

liberating and fun.

The reality is that porn is a harmful and addictive drug which hijacks your

natural healthy sexual instincts and exploits them for gain. The porn industry is not interested in sexual freedom, it is after profits.

And why do men get hooked? We get hooked because we are programmed to do so. Caveman is strongly visual and has powerful instincts to respond to the sight of a sexually attractive and available woman. In traditional cultures those drives would be triggered by real women – today it's the flood of cyberporn images. And so our natural Caveman instincts get bonded to an image on a screen rather than flesh and blood.

We stay hooked because addiction to porn is a distraction from unhappiness.

Behind most porn addiction is an emptiness. Loneliness, boredom, stress,

depression, feeling sexual disempowered, loss of direction in life, unexpressed

anger can all be fertile ground for a porn addiction to take root. Porn distracts us from what's missing in our life but it doesn't actually fill the emptiness. Men are drawn to porn because it seems to offer power, freedom and excitement. The reality is very different.

If you want to last longer in bed, if you want to stay harder and come much later, you only need to do one thing. I am sorry to break this to you, but porn has really ruined sex for many guys.You might think that porn is a great quick and cheap way to get off. The internet, after all, is flooded with full length porn videos. The problem is, once you have a live female in front of you and you are doing it, all that porn can really get to your head.

Porn screws up your expectations. Porn anchors your sexuality to an unrealistic fantasy image rather than to intimacy and sensuality with a real person. Porn is almost entirely visual. It closes off the other senses of touch, smell and taste, so important to sexuality. It takes a man out of his body. Porn focuses almost entirely on idealised images of the feminine, leading men to ignore the depth, complexity and beauty of their own sexuality. Porn leads to an emotional/erotic desensitisation, in which more and more extreme images are needed to create the same" thrill". Porn can make it hard for a man to function in an emotional and intimate relationship with a real woman. Porn leads to erectile dysfunction and premature ejaculation.

Try this. Go onto a porn site, one of the countless sites that offers a string of free clips and watch a few clips. Don't go for anything too weird and kinky, just some regular bonking. But take a step back and watch like a scientist, an

observer. Observe what is really going on. Analyse what beliefs and messages

the clips are putting across.

Is this gourmet sex? Is this about presence rather than performance?

First, notice that few clips last longer than ten minutes, and that includes the

preamble and foreplay (such as it is!). The thrusting bit is usually over pretty

quick. What message is that putting across?

And look at the way the guys are pumping away hard and fast from the moment they enter. Are you basing your expectations of yourself on how they perform? The clips are trying to suggest these guys have unbelievable stamina. Actually, they don't. Much of what you see is smoke and mirrors - clever cutting and editing.

Porn negatively impacts on our ability to last longer in bed and enjoy prolonged and satisfying sex in several ways.

■ It takes us out of our body and our senses and traps us in fantasy.

■ It makes it difficult for us to function sexually with real women.

■ It teaches a very limited and crude range of sexual expressions.

■ It implants totally unrealistic expectations as to what a man is capable of.

When you watch porn and you get off on porn, you are training yourself to get off based on your schedule. The problem is, when you have a real live female in front of you and you are having sex with her, you have to get off based on each other's schedule.

Sex is no longer about you. Porn is all about you. Porn is sex on demand, because you are having sex with yourself. To last longer in bed, and become a better lover, you need to get off porn totally.

What to do if you've got a serious thing going with porn?

First get real. Get your head out of the sand and fully accept where you are.

You've got to be able to say clearly to yourself "I've got a problem with porn".

Recognize how porn is messing up your life: time wasted, money, deception,

barriers to real intimacy. Perhaps the biggest way porn messes you up is that you are dishonouring yourself as a man. You deserve more in life and more sexually, than a furtive wank in front of a screen.

Stop blaming yourself and let go of shame. You are not sick. You are not weak

minded. You are not a pervert. For whatever reason you've been tricked. Your

sexual urges and your erotic desires (even the darker ones) are healthy and

natural. The worst thing you are guilty of is being conned. **The cure for porn addiction is simple: STOP DOING IT.**

9. Masturbate Once a Week.

I know this might sound like a contradiction to the advice I just gave without porn, but it makes sense. When you masturbate once a week without the aid of porn, you can feel more in control of your body. At the very least, you feel more aware of the patterns and signals your body sends out.

By being aware of the signals your body sends out, you can then mentally override them. You can stimulate yourself in such a way that you can come longer. Also, you can stimulate yourself in such a way that you can stay harder longer.

Masturbating once a week without the aid of porn is all about achieving a higher level of sexual self-awareness. Be in touch with what truly excites you, and form the right mental images so you can drag out ejaculation longer. The big payoff here is that the better you are at this, the more intense your climaxes are. If you are like the typical guy, you would think that the sooner you come, the better. You are basically just settling for crumbs. Why settle for crumbs when you can have a nice cake?

The best way to do that is to pay more attention to yourself when you are masturbating, so you can psychologically condition yourself for a very very intense and full orgasm.

10. Look After Yourself

Sex can be affected by stress, physical conditions like diabetes, medication, post childbirth. It is important to check with your doctor if your sex drive has changed significantly. There are often things that the GP can do to help.

Take care of yourself physically. Eating healthily, exercising, avoiding bad habits you do what you can to stay fit and active, able to enjoy a healthy sex life for as long as possible. Also, take care of yourself mentally. Be interested in current affairs, the latest films, what is happening locally. Keep your conversation fresh and interesting and you will feel more positive and upbeat, with lots of topics to discuss.

Good hygiene is also important in staying attractive to your partner; showering, looking after your teeth, wearing clean clothes, making an effort to dress nicely, especially for a date night together demonstrates respect for them and for the relationship.

Conclusion

Congratulations! you've reached the end of this guide. I hope that you've learned lots of valuable information and new tools for managing premature ejaculation. But let me clear: You've finished this book, but not your quest to get premature ejaculation under control.

The techniques I've described here take time, dedication, and most important practice. Just as there's no one treatment for premature ejaculation, there are also no quick fixes. You're on a path to a more satisfying sex life, but there will be bumps along the road. That's part of coping with a chronic, lifelong condition. It's a given that you'll make mistakes along the way.

So don't give up. Trust me when I tell you that it will get easier, that you can satisfy your partner, and that you can enjoy better sex yourself. But managing premature ejaculation is just like fighting any battle: You need a variety of weapons in your arsenal for best results. That's why what I've outlined here is crucial for success. With a positive attitude, the willingness to stick with the program through good and bad, and the tools necessary to address all aspects of the problem, you can manage, and ultimately overcome, premature ejaculation.

I wish you the best, and I know that your woman will feel her best from this day forward.